MAHATMA GANDHI ON HEALTH

Books by the same Author

- Complete Biography of Mahatma Gandhi (The) (In 3 Volumes)
- Gandhi in Modern World
- Inspiring Thoughts of Mahatma Gandhi: Gandhi in Daily Life
- Mahatma Gandhi on Ethics
- Mahatma Gandhi on Sarvodaya
- Mahatma Gandhi on Untouchability
- Mahatma Gandhi Speaks: Selected Speeches and Writings
- Revisiting HIND SWARAJ
- Understanding Gandhi: Speeches and Writings That Reveal His Mind, Methods and Mission
- World Crisis and the Gandhi Way
- Gaol Experiences of Mahatma Gandhi
- Gandhi and Nehru: Reflections Through Letters

About the Author

Anil Dutta Mishra is a distinguished Gandhian Scholar and Writer. He started his career as Assistant Professor in the Department of Non-violence and Peace Studies, Jain Vishva Bharati University, Ladnun, Rajasthan, became Deputy Director of National Gandhi Museum and Honorary Professor, Centre for Gandhian Philosophy and Human Development, Gayatri Vidya Parishad Degree College [Autonomous], Visakhapatnam. Presently, he is Treasurer, IIPA, Delhi Regional Branch, New Delhi.

Mishra has held the post of General Secretary of Indian Society of Gandhian Studies, Alliance for Sarvodaya, Member Board of Studies, Nagpur and Punjab Universities and is Member of Gandhian Studies Centre of different colleges and universities across India. He has authored/edited 30 books and published a number of research papers. His recent book **Reading Gandhi** is widely acclaimed.

Email: anilduttamishra@gmail.com

MAHATMA GANDHI ON HEALTH

Anil Dutta Mishra

CONCEPT PUBLISHING COMPANY PVT. LTD.
NEW DELHI-110059

ISBN-13: 978-93-5125-247-4

First Published 2016

Published and Printed by

Concept
Since 1974

Concept Publishing Company Pvt. Ltd.
Regd. Office:
A/15-16, Commercial Block, Mohan Garden,
New Delhi-110059 (INDIA)
Phones : 25351460, 25351794,
Fax : 091-11-25357109
Email : publishing@conceptpub.com
Website: www.conceptpub.com

Editorial Office: : H-13, Bali Nagar, New Delhi-110 015, India.

Cataloging in Publication Data—DK Courtesy: D.K. Agencies (P) Ltd. <docinfo@dkagencies.com>

Gandhi, *Mahatma,* 1869-1948., **author.**
Mahatma Gandhi on health / [translator], Anil Dutta Mishra.
pages cm
Translated from Gujarati.
Articles previously published in Indian opinion.
Includes index.
ISBN 9789351252474

1. Health. I. Mishra, Anil Dutta, 1965- translator. II. Title.

RA776.G36 2016 DDC 613 23

Preface

Gandhi during his stay in England and South Africa have acquired considerable experience, and have been able to form certain ideas on food and diseases to be cured. These ideas are may be of some use to the readers even in contemporary times. Gandhi believed that, *"Prevention is better than cure"*. *"The bund should be built before the flood"*. It is also true in case of health.

Gandhi gave much importance to health and hygiene. Like a lost jewel that takes greater effort to find than it does to keep it in the first instance, good health, once it is lost, costs much time and effort to regain. It is therefore essential for thoughtful people to attach the utmost importance to the keeping up of health. We shall consider further importance to the keeping up of health. We shall consider further how health, which may be lost from time to time, can be regained. It is the duty of everyone to understand the simple law of nature to keep oneself healthy.

While Gandhi was practicing law in South Africa he was suffering from digestive complaints. He used to take some herbal medicine. He thought that, every time taking some medicine for improving digestion and clearing bowels is not a proper way of treatment. He therefore thought that, there must be something wrong with the diagnosis and management of his problem. He was taking some medicines but they were ineffective. He thought that, what was the use of such therapy when every day one has to depend on a doctor and a chemist. One of his friend gave him a book "Return to the Nature" written by Adolf Just. He studied that book and tried simple measures like dietary reform, mud application over abdomen, use of wet compresses etc. He experienced relief by these simple measures. He thought that, such drugless therapy would be beneficial for India, where most of the people live in villages and they do not have access to doctors and hospitals. He wrote about his experiments in his own publication "Indian opinion" under the title "Guide to health" and some articles on nature cure, use of five elements and its effects. Those articles were written during the year 1906. When Gandhi returned to India, those compiled articles were published while he was confined in Aga Khan Palace in 1942. The book is known as "Key to Health". It is translated in different Indian and European languages. The book became popular because Gandhi wrote with a novel idea somewhat different from the ways adopted by medical practitioners and medical scientists.

Gandhi incorporated education in health and hygiene in his 18-point constructive programmes aimed at achieving complete independence by truthful and non-violent means. He emphasised on vegetarianism, which is inseparable from naturopathic way of treatment. He believed in his famous eleven vows namely *'Non-violence, Truth, Control over Palate (taste), Celibacy, Physical work, Non-stealing, Non-possession, Fearlessness, Removal of caste barrier, Equality in religion, Swadeshi or self-reliance.'*

"It is Health that is real Wealth and not pieces of gold and silver" Gandhi believes that modern medicine is the bane of man when used to perpetuate bad habits. Unpleasant reactions to food, drink or bad habits are our body's way of telling us to form better habits but instead we resort to medicine to mask the symptoms and inculcates faith in our body's own self-healing mechanisms.

Gandhi states that it is necessary to have knowledge about one's body which most of them are ignorant about. Human body is composed of five elements- Earth, Water, Vacancy, Light and Air. Good working of the human body depends upon the harmonious activity of the various component parts. The first element Air without which we can't live is surrounded us on all sides. Gandhi says that those who do not know how to breathe should take breathing exercises, further he gives the importance of cleaning the nostrils and the importance of sleeping under open sky. The second element Water which is basic necessity of life should be pure and it's the municipality's responsibility to provide clean water and to maintain the sewage and drainage system. The third element Earth which can be used as nature's way to treat ailments i.e., mud poultices to cue scorpion sting, constipation ordinary boils etc. The other element light which we get from sun has many uses such as sunbaths. The last vacancy, which can be also termed as Akash which helps to maintain and regain health.

Human body is composed of the five natural elements. Gandhi wrote about importance of five natural elements for maintaining health and in disease conditions. The concepts of eastern naturopathy differ from concepts of western naturopathy. Gandhi has given importance to all five elements whereas western naturopaths take into consideration only 4 elements. Scarcely the importance is given to psychological, moral and spiritual well being of individual and society. Gandhi was of the opinion that, the treatment should be very simple. Natural elements like Sun, Air, Earth, water and food available locally, physical labour (Shram) should be used for treatment of acute and chronic diseases.

Gandhi gave much importance to brahmacharya/celibacy which ultimately lead to a healthy life. It is the mode of life which leads to realization of God. The realization is through practicing self-restraint of senses. Gandhi rightly said that, "everything in the world can be used and abused and it applies to our body too. We abuse it when we use it for selfish purposes, in order to harm our body. It is put to right use if we exercise self-restraint and dedicate ourselves to the service of the whole world."

There are three categories of food: vegetarian, flesh and mixed. He believed that vegetarian is best among all followed by mixed. Gandhi states the importance of milk, cereals, pulses, fruits, vegetables, fats and the proportion in which it should be used. Regarding condiments Gandhi says, that body requires certain salts which mostly occur naturally in various food stuffs and from his personal experiments of fifty years is that there is no need for such condiments to keep body healthy except is necessary for medicinal purposes. Regarding sweets he is of the opinion that jaggery is the best among all and fried food should we avoided. Moving forward let us consider how often and how much to eat ? Gandhi said, "Food should be taken as a matter of duty even as a medicine to sustain the body, never for the satisfaction of palate. There should be self-control as such habits of elders influence children to some extent." The general rule is to take three meals.

The most important reason for illness in India is the defective and harmful method of answering calls of nature. The unhygienic toilets and defecating in open leads to major diseases. Hence, sanitation is a major problem. People are clean as individuals but not as members of society. In villages people bathe, wash clothes and drink water from same stream which is very unhygienic. Gandhi was quiet disturbed by the untidy sight of pilgrimage places in India. It is the work of municipalities and also common man to keep the surrounding clean. Also every religion stresses on the importance of cleanliness and Gandhi stated that Indians should imitate the western countries regarding cleanliness. For improving the conditions education in health and hygiene is must.

Gandhi used ancient wisdom in modern context. Indian philosophy based on Vedic scriptures says that, there should be balance between five motor organs and five sense organs. Our mental poise depends upon what we perceive through our sense organs. Therefore, right kind of perception through motor and sense organs is essential for the knowledge of space, air, fire, water and earth. Moderation in hearing, touch, vision, taste and smell, speech, thoughts, action, is necessary for balance of these elements in the human body. Health depends upon how one observes the laws of nature. If one is aware and practices self-discipline and good impression then only health can be maintained. Any deviation from the laws of nature which are omnipresent, will cause ill health.

Celibacy doesn't have reference only for seminal ejaculation, but it has a wider meaning of control over five sense organs, five motor organs and the eleventh sensory and motor function of mind. Therefore, moderation in all activities is necessary for celibacy during married life. One can see the ill effect of over indulgence in sensory and motor organs which has resulted in outbreak of HIV, AIDS, high prevalence of psychosomatic diseases, diseases of locomotors system respiratory problems, depression and stress and disturbed family relationship.

Gandhi's writings on General Knowledge about Health are reproduced here without any distortions and alterations so that the readers drew their own conclusions. I am sure that the book 'Mahatma Gandhi on Health' will open new vistas of research and proper understanding of Gandhi on this issue.

In writing this book I had received, over the years, very valuable help from friends. I am grateful to them. My family has always stood behind me in all my academic endeavours. My wife, Dr. Sweta Mishra, went through the final draft and provided her valuable inputs and insight.

Last but not the least, I am grateful to Shri Ashok Kumar Mittal of Concept Publishing Company Pvt. Ltd., for bringing out this book in present form and that too within record time.

Anil Dutta Mishra
anilduttamishra@gmail.com

Contents

Preface v

1. General Knowledge About Health-I 1
2. General Knowledge About Health-II 4
3. General Knowledge About Health-III 8
4. General Knowledge About Health-IV 10
5. General Knowledge About Health-V 13
6. General Knowledge About Health-VI 16
7. General Knowledge About Health-VII 19
8. General Knowledge About Health-VIII 23
9. General Knowledge About Health-IX 27
10. General Knowledge About Health-X 32
11. General Knowledge About Health-XI 38
12. General Knowledge About Health-XII 42
13. General Knowledge About Health-XIII 45
14. General Knowledge About Health-XIV 50
15. General Knowledge About Health-XV 54
16. General Knowledge About Health-XVI 59
17. General Knowledge About Health-XVII 63
18. General Knowledge About Health-XVIII 71
19. General Knowledge About Health-XIX 74
20. General Knowledge About Health-XX 78

21. General Knowledge About Health-XXI 82
22. General Knowledge About Health-XXII 85
23. General Knowledge About Health-XXIII 88
24. General Knowledge About Health-XXIV 91
25. General Knowledge About Health-XXV 94
26. General Knowledge About Health-XXVI 97
27. General Knowledge About Health-XXVII 99
28. General Knowledge About Health-XXVIII 103
29. General Knowledge About Health-XXIX 106
30. General Knowledge About Health-XXX 110
31. General Knowledge About Health-XXXI 113
32. General Knowledge About Health-XXXII 115
33. General Knowledge About Health-XXXIII 121

Index 125

1
General Knowledge About Health-I

I have had to reflect on the subject of health for the past twenty years. Having gone to England and having [earlier] become used to a particular mode of living, I had to devise my own arrangements for food. I can claim that, as a result, I have acquired considerable experience, and have been able to form certain ideas thanks to that experience. I write these chapters in the hope that they may be of some use to the readers of *Indian Opinion*.

There is a saying in English, "Prevention is better than cure".

"The bund should be built before the flood",[1] expresses a similar idea. Taking steps to prevent disease is, in English, termed "hygiene". In Gujarati, it may be called *Arogya Samrakshan Shastra*.

This science is distinct from medicine, though some take it to be a branch of medicine. My only reason for mentioning this distinction is that, in these chapters, the means for the care of health will be described for the most part. Like a lost jewel that takes greater effort to find than it does to keep it in the first instance, good health, once it is lost, costs much time and effort to regain. It is, therefore, essential for thoughtful people to attach the utmost importance to the keeping up of health. We shall consider further importance to the keeping up of health. We shall consider further how health, which may be lost from time to time, can be regained.

Milton, the English poet has observed that both Heaven and Hell exist only in the mind of man.[2] Hell does not lie underneath the earth, nor heaven in the clouds. This idea appears in Sanskrit literature, too. "The mind is the cause at once of bondage (hell) and *Moksha*[3] (heaven)." Pursuing this line of thought, we may argue that whether a person is ill or well he is himself for the most part responsible. One falls ill owing to one's thoughts as well as one's deeds. There are numerous instances of a father contracting cholera on seeing his son suffer from it. A distinguished physician has remarked that more patients die of fear than of the plague or other diseases. The saying that "a coward dies without being dead"[4] deserves to be pondered over.

Ignorance is also a great cause of broken health. When overtaken by misfortune, our ignorance makes us helpless, and we don't know what to do; with the best of intentions, we do the wrong thing.

Being unacquainted with the common rules concerning the human body, we often do things which we ought not to, or fall into the hands of selfish and unscrupulous quacks. It is surprising but true that we know less of things close by than of those that lie far away. I might be ignorant of the topography of my street but learn by heart the names of cities and rivers in England. I will patter away about the stars in the sky but you may be sure that I know nothing of the roof atop my house. I will think of country up the stars but do not ever feel the urge to know what there is in the roof above and how many rafters have gone to its making. I do not care to watch the drama that Nature enacts before my eyes but want to watch the got up shows in the theatre. In the same way, I have no knowledge of what happens in my body—what it is, what it is made of, how the bones, flesh and blood are formed, what their functions are, who it is within me that speaks, how my movement is affected, why I think good thoughts one moment and wicked ones at another, why my mind runs ten million miles away against my will, why, when my body moves at a snail's pace, my mind can move a thousand times swifter than the wind. I thus know less than nothing about the relation which my body, nearer to me than the nearest of things, has to my mind.

It is the duty of everyone to free himself from this predicament. To discover the relation between the body and the mind is an exacting task, but everyone should consider it essential to have some idea of the normal working of the human body. This knowledge should also form part of the education given to children. When one sits down to think about it, it is a matter for shame that, when my finger is cut, I should not know what to do about it, or, when pricked by a thorn, I should be unable to take it out or, upon being bitten by a snake, I cannot think of what to do at once without losing my nerve. To argue, using difficult words, that a layman cannoy understand these matters is sheer conceit, or worse still, a "fraud to exploit mankind".

We shall, with the help of these chapters, try and enable readers of *Indian Opinion* to free themselves, to some extent, of such dependence and ignorance, if they have not already done that.

Not that such articles have not been published elsewhere. People, however, get into the habit of reading particular books or newspapers.

The readers of *Indian Opinion* have come to read this journal along with a few others. Some of them do not read books on health. It is likely that they will benefit from the following chapters. Moreover, I intend, in these chapters, to provide an abstract of the views found in a number of books. I have read many books, considered contradictory opinions and, having put them to the test, have formed certain ideas.

Consequently, there will be found in these chapters the substance of more than one book. What is more, they will possibly spare the beginner the bewilderment caused by books that contradict one another. One book recommends the use of warm water for a particular condition while another suggests cold water. This may confuse the beginner. These contradictory courses of action will be considered in these chapters in the light of reason. Those who so desire may then refer to the original books and thus modify these conclusions. One may, therefore, safely assume that these chapters will prove useful, to a greater or lesser extent, to every reader of *Indian Opinion*.

[From Gujarati] *Indian Opinion*, 4-1-1913

NOTES

1. A Gujarati saying.
2. The mind is its own place, and in itself Can make a heav'n of hell, a hell of heav'n.
3. Liberation.
4. A Gujarati saying.

2
General Knowledge About Health-II

It is our habit that, at the slightest illness, we rush at once to a doctor, *vaidya* or *hakim*.[1] And if we do not, we take whatever medicine the barber or our neighbour suggests. It is our belief that no sickness can be cured without drugs. This, however, is sheer superstition.

People who suffer from other causes are—and will continue to be—fewer than those who have suffered, and are suffering, because of this superstition. If, therefore, we can get to know what constitutes illness, we should be able to take a somewhat balanced view. "*Darad*"[2] means pain. "*Roga*"[3] means much the same. It is right to seek a remedy for pain, but it is futile to take drugs to suppress pain. Actually, the result is often harmful. Taking medicine has the same effect as my covering up the refuse in my house. Refuse which is kept covered will putrefy and cause me harm. Moreover, the covering itself may putrefy and add to the refuse. I have then to get rid of the refuse which has since formed as well as that which was to begin with. This is the fate that befalls people taking drugs. But, if one throws out the refuse, the house will become as clean as it was before. By giving rise to illness—pain [that is]—Nature, in fact, informs us that there exists impure matter in our body. Moreover, Nature has provided within the body itself the means of cleansing it, so that, when illness occurs, we should realize that there exists impure matter in the body and that she has commenced her cleansing process. I should be thankful to anyone who came forward to remove the refuse from my house. So long as he has not done with the cleaning, I might be inconvenienced but I would keep my patience. Likewise, if I am patient while Nature is cleansing the body, which is my home, it will be well again, and I shall become healthy and so free from pain. If I have a cold, I do not have to rush to swallow drugs—*sunth*[4] [for instance]. I know that some impure matter has accumulated in a certain part of my body and that Nature has stepped in to remove it. And so I must let her have her way, so that my body may be cleansed in the shortest possible time. If I resist

Nature, her task is doubled; she has both to cleanse me and cope with my resistance. I can assist Nature, for instance, by getting rid of the effective cause of the impurity, so that more of it does not accumulate.

That is to say, if I stop eating for the duration of the illness, thus preventing the ingress of further impurity, and if I exercise in fresh air, I shall also start ejecting the impurity through the skin. That this is the golden rule for keeping the body free of disease, everyone can prove for himself. Only, the mind must be kept in a stable state. One who reposes true faith in God will always act in this fashion. The following [thought] will help in bringing about this state of mind:

'Even if I undergo the treatment prescribed by the *vaidya* or some such person, no one can guarantee that my disease will be got rid of.

Not all those who put themselves in the hands of a doctor are cured. If they were, Mr. Gandhi should not have to write these chapters and all of us would be leading happy lives.'

Experience shows that once the [medicine] bottle enters a house, it never leaves. Countless persons suffer from some ailment or other throughout their lives, go on adding to the drugs one after the other or go on changing their *vaidyas* and *hakims* in their search for the one who will cure them; finally, having ruined both themselves and others, they die, a troubled death. That famous judge, the late Mr. Justice Stephen, who had lived in India [for a time], once said that doctors introduce herbs, of which they know little, into bodies of which they know even less. Doctors say the same thing after attaining due experience.

Dr. Magendie has said: "Medicine is a great hoax." A famous doctor, Sir Ashley Cooper, has observed: "The science of medicine is based on mere guess-work." Sir John Forbes has remarked: "Notwithstanding the skill of physicians, it is Nature which cures most men of their diseases." Dr. Baker tells us: "In cases of night fever many more patients die of the drugs than of the disease." Dr. Froth declares that it is difficult to find a more dishonest profession than that of medicine. Dr. Thomas Watson writes: "In the most important matters our profession drifts on a sea of dubious hypotheses." Dr. Coswell feels that the human race would benefit immeasurably if the entire medical profession was ended. Dr. Frank avers that thousands have been killed in hospitals. Dr. Mason Good says: "Drugs claim a heavier sacrifice of human lives than do wars, epidemics and famines." We find that an increase in the number of doctors is followed in one place after another by a rise in the incidence of disease. Large advertisements appear in newspapers which do not accept other advertisements. When *Indian Opinion* used to accept advertisements, its workers had to go about soliciting these from others, but as for drug advertisements, their manufacturers pressed them on the journal and would even tempt [us] with large sums. We pay a rupee for medicine which should cost no more than a pie. Most manufacturers generally do not let us know what the drugs are made from. A drug-manufacturer recently brought out a book entitled *Secret Medicines*, his object being to ensure that people are not misled. He reveals therein that the ingredients of sarsaparilla, fruit salt, syrup and other well-known patent medicines, for which we pay from three to seven shillings a bottle, cost from a farthing to a penny. This means that we pay from 36 to 336 times the actual cost of the medicine. The profit to the dealer is thus 3500 to 35000 per cent.

The reader ought surely to see from all this that it is unnecessary for a patient to rush to a doctor or buy drugs in a hurry. But few will so forbear. All doctors are not dishonest. That every time the drug is harmful, the common man will not admit. To such persons, one may say: 'Forbear as much as you can. Do not bother a doctor as long as you can help it. If you must call in one, get only a reliable person and, having called him, stick to him. Consult another only if he so advises.

Your disease is not under your doctor's control. If it is given to you to live, you will get well and if, in spite of all that you have done, death comes to you or to your relatives, know that death is no more than a transition.' The purpose in my writing these chapters is that we might think and act according to this principle. In these, I wish to discuss with readers such topics as physiology, air, water, diet, exercise, clothing, water and earth treatment, accidents, child-care, the duties of men and women during pregnancy and common ailments.

MOHANDAS KARAMCHAND GANDHI
Phoenix
[From Gujarati] *Indian Opinion*, 11-1-1913

NOTES

1. A *vaidya* practices the Ayurvedic and *hakim* the Unani system of medicine.
2. Gujarati words for pain, ailment, disease.
3. *Ibid.*
4. Ginger, dried and ground, is a much used household remedy.

3
General Knowledge About Health-III

CHAPTER 1: THE HEALTHY STATE

It is the common belief that, if a person eats and drinks normally, moves about and does not call in the doctor, he is free from illness. A little thought will show that this belief is erroneous. Numerous instances come to notice of a person who eats, drinks and goes about and who ignores his ailments in the belief that there is nothing wrong with him.

In truth, there are very few persons in this world who are entirely healthy. An English writer has observed that only he can be called healthy in whose pure body dwells a pure mind. Man is not all body. The body is merely his abode. Moreover, the body, the mind and the sense-organs are so closely connected that, if one of them is affected by illness or pain, the others also get out of order. The body has been likened to a rose. What shows without is the body of the rose, the fragrance is its soul. No one would care for a paper rose which does not smell like the real flower. The fragrance is the test of the rose, so is the test of a man his fragrance—the character of his soul. We will, moreover, throw away a flower which looks like a rose but has an unpleasant smell. Likewise, even if a man's body appears to be all right, if the soul inhabiting that body tends to bad conduct, his body will hold no fascination for us. We thus see that one whose character is unworthy can never be called healthy. The body is so closely bound to the soul that one whose body is pure will be pure in mind too. In the West a whole tradition has emerged, based on this principle. It holds that those whose minds are pure can never be ill and one who is ill can cure himself by cultivating purity of mind. this tenet should not be rejected [out of hand]. It is sound, in fact, but the people of the West who claim to be civilized misuse it. The essential thing we have to learn from this tradition is that our mind is a potent means for the preservation of health, and that purity of mind ensures the maintenance of good health.

This man has a bad temper and is *tamasik*[1], that man is lethargic.

A third is deaf. All these defects are, in fact, only symptoms of disease. Some doctors believe that even faults, such as stealing, are diseases. Some wealthy women in England pilfer worthless articles from shops. Doctors in that country ascribe this state of mind to a disease termed kleptomania. There are a few who are not at peace till they have shed blood. This, too, is a disease.

Arguing along these lines, we can describe only that person as healthy whose body is whole and without defect; whose teeth are sound; who has his ears and eyes; whose nose does not run; who does perspire but whose perspiration does not smell; whose feet and mouth do not give out a bad odour; whose hands and feet can perform common tasks; who is not given to inordinate sexuality; who is neither too fat nor too thin, and whose mind and senses are under control. It is no easy matter to achieve or maintain this state of health. We do not enjoy such good health because our parents did not. A great writer has said that the offspring, if any, of men and women who are fit in every way must surpass their parents. If this be untrue, those who hold that the world is progressing must revise their view. One who is wholly free from disease has no fear of death. The very fact that we all fear death shows that we are not healthy. Death is for us a great transformation and, according to the law of creation, should be a noble one. It is our duty to strive for this lofty kind of health. How such health can be gained and preserved, we shall inquire hereafter.

[From Gujarati] *Indian Opinion*, 18-1-1913

NOTE

1. Full of darkness.

4
General Knowledge About Health-IV

2. OUR BODY

Earth and water, sky, fire and air.
The play of these five elements, they call the Universe.

An almost full description of the human body is contained in this verse. It says that the sport of Nature or her Creator with the five elements—earth, water, sky, light and air—which he mingles, is what we know by the name of the Universe. From the substance of which this Universe is made has been fashioned this figure of clay which we call our body. We have a saying among us, "as within the body so in the Universe"[1] and, "as with oneself, so with the country". If we remember this clue [to the mystery of the Universe] we shall certainly see that clean earth, pure water, fresh air and open space and bright sunshine are essential for the preservation of the body, and that we need not fear any of these elements. In fact, illness follows when the body becomes comparatively deficient even in one of these. It is imperative that we know at least this much about our body, but this knowledge is not adequate for our subject.

The body is made up of skin, bone, flesh and blood. The skeleton provides the principal support for the body and it is that which enables us to stand upright and walk. The bones protect the delicate parts of the body, the skull protects the brain and the ribs, the heart and the lungs. There are 238 bones in the body by the doctors' reckoning. We can all see that a bone is hard outside, but it is not so inside; the inside is soft and hollow. The joint where one bone is joined to another is covered with cartilage which is taken to be soft bone.

Our teeth, too, are bones. During childhood, the milk-teeth first appear and these fall out. Then permanent teeth appear, which, once they drop out, do not grow again. Milk-teeth begin appearing between the ages of six and eight months and have almost all of them appeared by the time the child is about two years old. Permanent teeth begin to appear after the age of five and they have all grown by the time he is between seventeen and twenty-five. The molars appear last of all.

If we feel our skin, we will find a number of knobs of flesh underneath at many places. These are called muscles. Our nerves get work out of them. It is because of our muscles that we can open and close our hands, work our jaws and blink. All these actions are performed with the aid of muscles.

Complete information about the body lies outside the scope of these chapters. The writer himself does not possess this knowledge.

Only facts necessary for our purpose will be set out here. Having, therefore, grasped the foregoing facts, we go on to the main parts of the body. Among these, the stomach is the most important. If the stomach were to slacken even for a moment, all our limbs would languish. Even the most ferocious beast will not have the capacity to endure the strain which we subject the stomach to. Its function is to digest food and nourish the body with the food so assimilated. What the engine is to machinery, the stomach is to man. This organ is to the left, beneath the ribs. Having passed through many processes within it, the food is then broken down into different fluids and their [nutritive] element extracted, the remaining portion being expelled from the intestines as excreta. Above the stomach is the left lobe of the liver. To the left of the stomach is the spleen. The liver is to the right beneath the ribs. Its function is to purify the blood and produce bile which is needed for the digestive process.

Behind the ribs, in the hollow of the chest, are [located] other useful organs—the heart and the lungs. The sac containing the heart is to the left, between the two lungs. There are altogether 24 bones in the chest including both those to the left and to the right. The heart pulsates between the fifth and the sixth ribs. We have tow lungs, the left and the right, which consist of bronchial tubes. These are filled with air and purify the blood. Air reaches the lungs through the windpipe.

This air must pass through the nostrils. Air which thus passes through the nostrils is warmed before it reaches the lungs. Many people, who are ignorant of the fact, breathe through the mouth and so do themselves harm. The mouth is for eating, etc. Air must be inhaled only through the nose.

We have briefly examined the structure of the body and got some idea of its important parts. Now we shall examine the fluid—blood—on which the functioning of our body depends. Blood provides us with nourishment. It separates the nutritive part of the food, expels the useless products—excreta—and maintains the body at a constant temperature. It flows continuously through veins and arteries. It is to this flow that the pulse-beat is due. In a young and healthy person the pulse beats about 75 times a minute. A child's pulse is more rapid and that of an aged person slower.

The most important agent that keeps the blood pure is air. The blood which enters the lungs, having circulated through the body, has become useless as it now contains poisonous substances. The air inhaled into the lungs absorbs these toxic substances and passes on the oxygen it contains to the blood stream. This process goes on constantly. The inhaled air, laden with the poisons from the blood, then comes out and the blood, having taken up the oxygen, circulates through the arteries over the entire body. One can imagine the extent to which the exhaled breath is impure. Air has such tremendous effect on our bodies that it will be necessary to consider the subject in some detail in a separate chapter.

[From Gujarati] *Indian Opinion*. 25-1-1913

NOTE

1. The saying is, "...".

5
General Knowledge About Health-V

3. AIR

We have seen something of the structure of the body and have learnt that it requires three kinds of nourishment: air, water and food.

Of these, air is the most essential. Consequently, Nature has provided it to such extent that we can have it at no cost. But modern civilization has put a price even on air. In these times, one has to go off to distant places to take the air, and this costs money. It is at Matheran that residents of Bombay can get fresh air and only then does their health improve. In Bombay itself, if one can live on Malabar Hill, the air is much better. But one must have money to do this. If Durbanites want fresh air, they have to go to live in Berea. That again means expense.

It would not, therefore, be quite true to say in modern times that "air is free".

Whether air is free or has to be paid for, we cannot carry on without it for a moment. We have seen that blood circulates through the entire body, is purified after returning to the lungs and flows out again. This goes on all day and all night. Every time we breathe out, we expel fouled air and, when we breathe in, we obtain from the air without, oxygen with which to purify the blood. This respiration continues every moment and the life of our body depends upon it. When we die of drowning, it only means we are unable to inhale oxygen and exhale foul air. A pearl diver puts on a diving suit before he goes down into the water and obtains air from a tube [one end of] which remains above the water-level. It is because of it that he can remain under water for a long time.

Some doctors have conducted experiments which have established that, if a person is kept without air for five minutes, the life giving breath leaves the body. At times a baby [lying] close to its mother dies of suffocation. This happens because the mouth and nose are smothered, and the baby gets no fresh air.

We see from all this that air is the most necessary nourishment for us, one that can be had without the asking. We get food and water, only by asking for or seeking them, but air, we take in involuntarily.

Just as we hesitate to take foul water or food, so ought we to in the case of foul air. In fact we do not take in unwholesome food or polluted water in the same quantities as we do in case of foul air. The revulsion comes from the seeing. [For] we worship idols.[1] Air cannot be seen with the naked eye. We, therefore, have no idea of how much foul air we take in. We hesitate to eat food touched by another; we would think twice before drinking water which another has tasted before us. Even if we felt no aversion[2] within us [towards filth or ugliness], we would never take the vomit of another. If vomit is put even before one famine-stricken, he would die rather than eat it. But we all inhale, without revulsion, the air "spewed" by another—that is, exhaled by him. According to the rules of hygiene, spewed air is just as bad as spewed food. It has been proved that, if air exhaled by a man is introduced into the lungs of another, the latter dies instantaneously; so poisonous it is. Yet people sitting of sleeping cooped up in a small room inhale, all the time, air which is as impure.

Fortunately, air is constantly in a state of movement and agitation and diffuses rapidly. Moreover, it can enter through the smallest of pores.

Consequently, even as we are huddled in a room and fouling the air inside, some fresh air comes through a clearance in the door or chinks in the roof. It is not wholly "spewed" air, therefore, that we [they] breathe. The air exhaled by us is constantly being purified. When we breathe the air inside us out into the open, the foul air diffuses instantly into the atmosphere, and Nature thus maintains the [required] quantity of pure air. The atmosphere extends over a large area, enveloping this small earth.

We can now see why so many people are ailing and emaciated.

There is no doubt *that bad air is the cause of more than 99 per cent of diseases*. Tuberculosis, fever and many diseases termed infectious are all caused by the foul air we inhale. The first, the easiest and the last means of ending them is to have fresh air, purest of the pure.

There is no other, *vaidya or hakim*, that can match it. Tuberculosis is a sign of rotting lungs, foul air being the cause. Just as an engine is damaged through being fed with bad coal, so are our lungs by foul air. Hence, modern doctors who understand [this] will invariably advise tuberculosis patients, as the first step in the treatment, to spend all the 24 hours in the open. All other remedies take effect after this, but none will work without it.

[From Gujarati] *Indian Opinion*, 1-2-1913

NOTES

1. That is, we believe only in good or evil that is visible.
2. For the same concept, *vide* "Nausea", 2-2-1907.

6
General Knowledge About Health-VI

We consume air not only with the lungs, but some portion of it is also taken in through the skin. On the skin, there are pores, minute and innumerable, through which we draw air.

Everybody ought to know how a thing so essential may be kept clean. Indeed, as soon as a child's understanding is adequate, he should be taught about the importance of air. If the readers of these chapters perform this easy but important task and, having acquired some general knowledge about air, live according to it, pass on the knowledge to their children and make them act in accordance, I shall regard myself as having fulfilled my task.

Latrines, open spaces, narrow lanes [dirtied through misuse] and urinals, where these are separate, are the principal agencies for defilement of air. Few are aware of the harm that can be caused by the filth from latrines. When a cat or dog defecates, it generally paws a hole and, having defecated into it, covers the faeces over with earth.

Where modern water-closets do not exist, this method ought to be followed. We should keep a pail full of dry earth or ash in our latrines. Every time the latrine is used, earth or ash should be sprinkled over the faeces so as to cover them over completely. This will stop the smell, and it cannot then happen that flies and winged insects, having sat on the filth, come in contact with our bodies. One whose nose has not become defective or injured to stench can easily realize how much foul odour, filth kept uncovered can spread. If filth from a latrine were mixed in our food in our presence, we should be sick. But there is not an iota of difference between air laden with the stench from a latrine and food mixed with faeces. If there is, it is only that the latter is visible to our naked eye, while the former is not. Seats, etc., in closets should be kept absolutely clean. We are ashamed to do this kind of work ourselves, or fret at having to do it, instead of which we should feel disgust at having to use dirty latrines. Why should we not ourselves clean up the filth excreted by our own body, which we make another person take away? There is absolutely nothing bad about doing this work oneself; having learnt this for ourselves, we must teach it to our children as well. When the pail is full, the contents should be thrown into a pit, a foot or two deep, and should be well covered over with earth. If one is in the habit of going to the fields to defecate, one should go far from where people live. There, one should dig a shallow pit with a spade to get one's business over with and should fully cover the faeces with the earth dug.

We urinate any and everywhere and this fouls the air; it is a habit that must be wholly given up. Where no special place is available for urination, we should go far from where people live; having made water on dry ground, we should sprinkle the spot with earth. There are forceful reasons, however, why excreta should not be buried too deep.

One is that the heat of the sun cannot then do its work and the second that it may affect the neighbouring springs.

We spit on the carpet, on the floor, in the courtyard and wheresoever we can. Spittle is often poisonous. The sputum of a tubercular patient is extremely dangerous. Germs rising from it get into the air inhaled by others and do great harm. Over and above that, the house is dirtied, but that is another matter. In this regard our duty is not to spit any and everywhere inside the house, but to keep a spittoon.

Outdoors, one should spit, if one has to, on dry ground where there is plenty of dust. The sputum will mix with the dry earth and the damage will be less. Some doctors are of the opinion that tubercular patients should spit only into receptacles containing germicide. Even if a patient spits onto the dust on dry ground, the germs in his sputum are not destroyed. This dust carrying the germs rises into the atmosphere and infects others. Whether this opinion is right or wrong, we can at least learn this much from it: spitting any and everywhere is a dirty and injurious habit.

Some people are in the habit of throwing food, refuse and peelings, etc., all over. If this garbage was buried in the ground near the surface, it would not foul the air; also it would in due course make useful manure. One should never throw out perishables. It has been found from experience that these suggestions are easily put into practice, once they are understood.

We have seen how air is fouled through our bad habits and how this can be stopped. We shall now consider how it should be inhaled.

[From Gujarati] *Indian Opinion,* 8-2-1913

7
General Knowledge About Health-VII

We saw in the previous chapter that the correct way of inhaling air is through the nose—not the mouth; few really know how to breathe correctly. Many people breathe through the mouth. This habit is injurious. If very cold air is inhaled through the mouth, one catches a cold and the voice drops. Dust particles in the air enter the lungs of one who breathes through the mouth and they often do much damage. One immediately experiences this at first hand in a large city like London. Thanks to the large number of chimneys, frequent "fogs"—yellow mists—form in that city in November. Minute black particles are suspended in the fog. They will be found in the sputum of one who inhales air laden with this dust. To avoid this happening, some women, who are not accustomed to breathing through the nose, tie a gauze mask over their mouths. This gauze serves as a kind of strainer. The air passing through it is cleared. If this mask is examined after use, these particles are seen. God has placed a similar filter in our nose. Air breathed in through the nose reaches the lungs only after it has been cleansed.

Moreover, this air goes down after it has been warmed. Keeping these facts in mind, everyone should learn to breathe in only through the nose. This is no difficult matter. When we are not talking, the mouth should be kept shut. Those who have got into the habit of leaving their mouths open should sleep at night with a bandage over the mouth. Breathing then will necessarily be through the nose. One should also take about 20 deep breaths through the nose, morning and evening, standing in the open. By so doing the habit of breathing through the nose is formed.

Even if a healthy person who is accustomed to breathing through the nose does this, his chest will become strong and broad. This experiment should be tried by everyone. One should measure one's chest before commencing this experiment and again a month later. One will find that the chest has become appreciably broader even in so short a period. Sandow and others get people to exercise with dumb-bells, and the principle underlying it is the same. Exercising briskly with dumb-bells makes one breathe hard and deep. And this makes the chest broad and strong.

Together with the knowledge of how to breathe, it is also necessary to develop the habit of inhaling fresh air day and night. Our normal custom is to remain confined in our house or shop by day, and at night to sleep in a room that is like a safe. If the room has doors and windows, we shut them. *This habit must be strongly deprecated.*

It is imperative that we inhale pure air for as long as possible, especially while sleeping. Everyone who can manage to do so should accordingly sleep in an open veranda or on the terrace, outside the house or on the balcony. Those who do not have the good fortune to be able to do this should keep as many doors and windows open as possible. There is no need to fight shy of air, which is our staple diet twenty-four hours of the day. The notion that the fresh or raw air of morning causes illness is a mere superstition. It is possible that one who has spoiled his lungs through bad habits may contract a cold by sudden contact with fresh air, but one should not be afraid of this cold. In Europe, at various places, they have now put up, for persons suffering from tuberculosis, spacious buildings, which admit plenty of fresh air. The chief cause of the pestilence of plague in our own country is our bad habit of fouling the air and inhaling this defiled air. That even the most delicate of persons can only benefit from fresh air is a certain truth. If we learn not to foul the atmosphere and to take in only fresh air, we will, without any effort on our part, be spared many diseases, and the charge of slovenliness made against us in lands such as South Africa will to some extent be obviated.

Just as it is needful to sleep in the open, so it is not to cover one's face during sleep. It is the habit of many Indians to sleep with their faces covered. By so doing, we inhale the foul air we have exhaled. Air is a thing that finds its way through the smallest of passages. However, we muffle ourselves, some air does get in. If this did not happen, we would die of asphyxiation whenever we sleep covered right up to the head. But this does not happen, since some air from without, with oxygen in it, does enter; however, that is not enough. If one feels cold in the head, one can cover it separately as with a Balaclava cap, leaving the nose uncovered. However, cold it may be, one should never sleep with the nose covered.

Air and light are so closely connected that a word or two must be said about light in this chapter itself. As we cannot live without air, so we cannot do without light. Hell is conceived as absence of light.

Where there is no light, the air is always unwholesome. When we enter a dark room, we are bound to become aware of the smell. We cannot use our eyes in the dark; and this proves that we are born to live in the light. The darkness that Nature has thought necessary for us, she has given us by creating the comfort-giving night. Many people have got into the habit of sitting or sleeping, on the hottest of days, in cellar like rooms, having shut out light and air. Those who live without air and light look weak and lustreless.

In Europe nowadays, some doctors cure their patients by prescribing plenty of light and fresh air. It is not only the face that they expose to light and air; the patient is almost stripped and they then bring fresh air and light to play on the skin all over the body.

Hundreds of persons are cured by this treatment. In order to allow light and air to enter and leave freely, the windows of the house should be kept open day and night.

On reading this, people will wonder how it is that, if light and air are so necessary, many who remain confined to their rooms do not suffer any harm. It must be said that those who entertain this doubt have not thought about the matter. Our subject is not how to exist anyhow, but how to live, if possible, in perfect health. It has been conclusively proved that, where people get insufficient air and light, they are unwell all the time. City-dwellers are more delicate than village folk because they get less light and air. Among our people in Durban, diseases such as tuberculosis are prevalent and the Medical Officer ascribes it to the fact that we live in such conditions that we either cannot get or do not take in fresh air. The subject of air and light has so close a relation to good health that one should pay great attention to understanding it.

[From Gujarati] *Indian Opinion,* 15-2-1913

8
General Knowledge About Health-VIII

4. WATER

We have seen earlier that air is food. The same is true of water.

Air enjoys the first position, and water comes second. Without air man can survive only for a few minutes, whereas, he can live without water for hours, even for days on end, depending on the country. Even so, it is certain that one cannot subsist without water for as long as one can without food. If, however, a person can have water, he can live for many days without food. Water makes up more than 70 per cent of our body. Without water, it is believed, the body would weigh 8 to 12 lbs. In all that we eat, there is more or less water.

Yet we take proportionately little care of a thing which, for us, is very important. Diseases like the plague beset us because of our carelessness in the mater of air. Similar results follow from our carelessness regarding water. Typhoid often breaks out among troops in battle and the cause, it has been proved, is polluted water, because on the front soldiers have to drink whatever water they can get.

Typhoid breaks out also among those who live in cities, and the cause is mostly bad water. Drinking bad water often gives rise to diseases like stone.

There are two causes for contamination of water—one, that the water is found in places where it cannot remain pure, and two, that we sully the water. We ought not to drink water which is stores in or comes from a dirty place, and for the most part, we do not; but we do not hesitate to drink water which has been polluted by us through neglect. For instance, we throw whatever we like into a river and then proceed to use that very water for drinking and washing. The rule is that one should never drink water from the place where one bathes.

River-water should be drawn from a spot up stream where no one bathes. In every village, therefore, the river should be divided into two sections—the lower section for bathing and washing and the upper for drinking. When an army camps in the vicinity of a river, the direction of the river-flow is ascertained and a flag put up [at a given spot] on the bank. Anyone who bathes in a place higher up is punished. Where, in our country, these arrangements do not exist, careful women dig pits in the river-bed and take water from these; this practice is very wholesome as the water gets filtered as it passes through the sand.

Well-water is sometimes dangerous to drink. In shallow wells, the liquid from the excreta absorbed into the surrounding ground seeps in and pollutes the water. Sometimes dead birds fall into them; often birds build their nests within. Moreover, if there is no masonry round the well [at the top], dirt from the feet of persons drawing water falls into the well and fouls the water. It is therefore necessary to employ the utmost care in using well-water for drinking. Water stored in tanks is oftentimes bad. To prevent deterioration of such water, the tanks should be cleaned from time to time and kept covered; the roof and other places from where [drinking] water comes should be kept clean. Few, however, make the effort to maintain such cleanliness. The golden rule is therefore to rid the water of impurities to the extent possible; to boil it for half an hour; to let it stand for a time; to pour it into another vessel without disturbing the water and then to drink it only after straining it through thick, clean cloth into a third vessel.

One who does this is, however, not released from his duty towards others. Water which is maintained for public use is in the nature of property which jointly belongs to him and to all others living in the locality. He is obliged to use it like a trustee. He must, therefore, do nothing which might foul the water in any way. He must never foul a river or well. He must not bathe or wash clothes near any source of drinking water or defecate in the vicinity. He may not cremate dead bodies nearby or throw the ashes into the water.

Even after taking these precautions, we do not get water that is perfectly pure. It contains a certain amount of salts and, occasionally, rotten vegetable matter. Rain water is regarded as the purest of all, but before it reaches us the dust particles, etc., in the atmosphere get mixed with it. Absolutely pure water has a different effect on the body. Knowing this, certain doctors prescribe distilled water for their patients. This water is made by boiling water into steam and cooling the latter. Anyone suffering from constipation may, if he chooses, have first-hand proof of the efficacy of distilled water. Such water is sold by all chemists. A book has recently been published on the subject of distilled water and its uses. The writer believes that a large number of diseases can be cured by the use of water so processed.

This is an exaggeration, but it is not improbable that absolutely pure water has considerable effect on the body.

Not everyone knows that water is of two kinds, hard and soft; but the fact is noteworthy. Hard water is that in which soap does not readily lather but remains insoluble. This means that the water contains salts in large quantities. It is difficult to use soap with hard water, as it is with brackish water. With hard water, cooking too is difficult and, for the same reason, drinking it should, and does, make it difficult for us to digest our food. Hard water always tastes brackish whereas soft water is either sweet or tasteless. Some believe that, as the substances dissolved in hard water are nutritive, its use is beneficial, but we generally find that soft water is the right one to use. Rain is Nature's purest form of water. It is of course soft and all agree it is good to use. If hard water is boiled on a *chulha* for half an hour, it becomes soft. After it is taken off the fire, it should be processed as described earlier.

When to drink water and how much—the question sometimes arises. The simple answer to this is that water should be drunk when one feels thirsty and enough to quench one's thirst. There is nothing wrong in drinking water during or after a meal. Those who drink in the course of a meal should, however, remember that water is not to be drunk for washing down the food. If food does not go down by itself, that is either because it has not been properly chewed or because the stomach does not need it.

In fact, it is not—and it should not be—generally necessary to drink water. Just as our bodies consist of over 70 per cent of water, so does our food. In some foods, the proportion of water far exceeds 70 per cent. There is no food that is wholly devoid of water. Furthermore, much water is used in cooking. Why then does one feel thirsty? A complete answer to this question can be had only by reference to the constituents of our diet. Here, it may be simply said that those whose diet does not contain things like spices and chillies, which create an unnatural thirst, need only a little water. Those whose diet consists mainly of fresh fruit will seldom want to drink water by itself. If a person is constantly thirsty without reason, we may take it that he suffers from something or the other.

One notices that some people drink water indiscriminately, having superficially observed others doing so without any apparent ill-effects. The answer that was given to a similar question in the chapter on air applies here also. Moreover, the blood in our body possesses such wonderful properties that it destroys a number of toxins itself. But a fine sword is damaged if not burnished after use, and so with blood. If we get blood to do the work of a watchman, but do not look after it, it is not surprising that its power is sapped and finally lost altogether. Thus, if one always drinks bad water, the blood will in the end certainly stop doing its work.

[From Gujarati] *Indian Opinion*, 22-2-1913

9
General Knowledge About Health-IX

5. DIET

Air, water and food constitute our nourishment. But as a rule we look upon food alone as nourishment, and by food we only mean foodgrains. We will not believe that a person lives on food unless he eats wheat and rice.

The truth is that air is the principal form of nourishment. We have seen that we just cannot exist without it, also that we are taking in this essential form of nourishment every moment, whether we are aware of it or not. Water comes next in importance to air but before food, and so nature has seen to it that this also is more readily available than food. Food occupies the third and last place.

Food is unite a complicated subject to write on. There is much difference of opinion regarding what food to take and when. Habits differ from nation to nation. The same item of food affects different individuals differently. It is difficult, even impossible, to be dogmatic in this matter. In certain parts of the world men kill human beings and eat their flesh; for them it is food. There are also some who eat excreta. That is food for them. Some live entirely on milk; for them milk is food. Others, again, live on fruit and for them that is food. In this chapter the term "food" covers all these things. Although, it is difficult to lay down what food should be eaten, it is necessary for each one to come to some decision for himself. It is of course superfluous to observe that the body cannot function without food. We are ready to suffer innumerable hardships, even commit sins, in order to obtain food. Under these circumstances it is necessary to inquire into the purpose of taking food. We shall then be able to determine what food we should take. All will agree that out of every 100,000 persons 99,999 eat merely to please their palate, even if they fall ill in consequence. Some take a laxative every day in order to be able to eat well, or some powder to aid digestion. Some, having gorged an enormous meal with great relish, vomit it out and are ready again for other delicacies. Some eat large quantities and then miss a couple of meals. Some die of thoughtless overeating. The author has himself come across all these types. There has been such a transformation in his own life that he can now laugh at many of his past follies and is ashamed of some others. There was a time when the author would drink tea in the morning, have breakfast two or three hours later, a regular meal at one p.m., then tea at about three O'clock and a full meal between 6 and 7 in the evening. His condition in those days was pitiable indeed. He used to get oedema. A medicine bottle was always at his side. He would often have a laxative in order to be able to eat, and afterwards a dose from another bottle by way of tonic, as a matter of routine. He feels that he now has three times the energy for work that he then had, although he must be said to be no longer in his prime. Such a life is indeed to be pitied, and is if we go deeper into the matter, low, sinful and despicable.

Man is not born merely to eat, nor does he live merely for the sake of eating. He is born in order to know his Maker and he lives to this end. This cannot be done unless one keeps one's body alive and the latter cannot exist without food. This is why food is a necessity.

This is the ideal attitude and it will do for those who believe in God. But even the atheist will admit that one must eat with due regard to one's health and with the object of keeping the body fit.

Consider beasts and birds. Cattle do not eat for the satisfaction of the palate, nor do they eat like gluttons. They eat when they are hungry—and just enough to satisfy that hunger. They do not cook their food. They take their portion from that which Nature proffers to them. Then, is man born to pander to his palate? Is he alone fated to be always ill? Among the animals which are not domesticated, there is no starvation;

they have no rich and poor, nor is there one group that eats ten times in a day and another that can scarcely eat even once. All these distinctions are to be found only in our species, yet we regard ourselves as superior in intelligence to animals. It is, however, evident from all this, that if we make our stomach our God and spend our lives in its worship, we must surely be inferior to them.

If we think carefully, we shall discover that the root cause of the many evil things that we do, such as lying, pleasure-hunting, perjury, theft and so on, is our failure to restrain the craving of our palate. If we could keep it under control, we would find it easy enough to rid ourselves of the other cravings. In spite of our knowing this, we fail to regard over-eating or taking too much pleasure in food as a sin. If we steal or fornicate or tell a lie, others regard us with contempt. Among books on ethical subjects, many fine ones have been written on lying, stealing, adultery, etc., but there is no book about the kind of person who cannot control his palate. This subject is not, as a matter of fact, considered as falling under ethics. The reason for this is that we are, all of us, in the same boat. How will the pot call the kettle black? Even our great men do not appear to have succeeded in mastering the desire for tasty food. Consequently, indulging one's palate has never been considered to be wrong. The most that books recommend is that, in order to control the senses, it is desirable to limit the amount of food eaten. But it has never been said that the pampering of our palate makes us prone to other weaknesses as well. Thieves, cheats and sensual men are shunned by respectable people. But these same respectable people must be indulging in pleasures of the palate hundreds of times more varied than those of ordinary men and women. *A man's gentlemanliness is supposed to consists in the richness of his meals*. Thus, just as in a thieves' settlement stealing would not be a sin, so we, being all of us slaves of the palate, do not frown upon such slavery or even notice it. On the contrary, we are happy with it. At a wedding we give feasts to minister to the pleasures of the palate, our own and those of others. Some give dinners at funerals, too. On festival days, there must be sweets. When a guest comes, tasty dishes must be prepared. Not to invite neighbours and friends to partake of meals and not to go to them for the same purpose is frowned upon as grossly unsocial conduct. Unless we press the invited guest to overeat, we are considered to be extremely stingy.

On every holiday, we feel bound to prepare special dishes. On Sundays, we seem to think that we have the right to eat till we are sick.

What is, therefore, in the nature of a great fault has been transformed by us into an essential social obligation. The serving of meals is accompanied with numerous formalities of hypocritical nature, so that our slavery, our animality is completely hidden from ourselves. How shall we free ourselves from this darkness? This problem lies beyond the scope of simple hygiene. We can, therefore, only pose it and leave it there; it must be considered, however, to the extent that it bears on the problem of health.

Let us now look at the subject from another angle. It appears to be a universal law that the food needed by living creatures, whether human or animal, is provided by Nature from day to day. There is nothing strange in this. In Nature's kingdom no insurance is required.

No one is found remiss in his duty, none sleeps, no one is lazy. The water-wheel of her processes is in perpetual motion without so much as a moment's pause. And so Nature does not have to lay by a store for a year or even for a day. By this inexorable law are we governed, whether we wish it or no. If we understand and abide by it, not a single family will have to starve even for a day. Now, it is obvious that, if just sufficient food is produced every day and if one person eats more than his share—eats more than he needs, there is bound to be a shortage to that extent, and, therefore, insufficient food for another.

This is the simple explanation why large numbers of people have to go without food. In God's creation, in the kitchens of thousands of kings and hundreds of thousands of rich men, food is prepared that is far in excess of what they and their servants need. This excess has been taken out of the mouths of others. Will not these others then go hungry? If two wells are served the same current of water, and if this current carries just sufficient water for the two, it is quite plain that an excess of flow into one will mean shortage for the other. If this rule is correct—a rule which is not a figment of the author's imagination but one which has been propounded by highly intelligent men—it means that, whatever we eat after our hunger has been satisfied is stolen food.

Akha[1], the goldsmith, has truly sung: "Like unto unprocessed mercury swallowed in place of food is wealth stolen from another." Whatever we eat for the sake of its taste alone is to be paid for by the body through toxic reactions, either visible or invisible; we lose our health to that extent and suffer. After this discussion, it will be easier for us to consider what and when to eat.

[From Gujarati] *Indian Opinion,* 1-3-1913

NOTE

1. A Gujarati poet of the 17th century.

10
General Knowledge About Health-X[1]

In considering what food we should eat, let us first ask what we should not eat. If we designate as food all that enters the body byway of the mouth, then alcohol, cigarettes, tobacco, hemp, tea, coffee, cocoa, spices—all are food.

All these should be avoided. The author has found this to have been borne out by experience. Some of these articles he has consumed himself; regarding the rest he has observed the experience of others.

It is necessary to write about alcohol and hemp. All religions regard them as bad. There is hardly anyone who will defend their consumption. Alcohol has brought destruction to entire families.

Millions of drunkards have been ruined. Under the influence of drink a man ceases to be himself. Such a one sometimes forgets the difference between mother and wife. This vice corrodes the intestines and, in the final stages, the victim becomes a burden upon the earth. Drunkards may be seen rolling in the gutters. A respectable man turns into a man of straw when he gets drunk. It is not that a person falls into such a state only when he drinks. An alcohol addict, one will observe, is feeble-minded even when sober. He has no control over his mind, which wanders like a child's. Alcohol, as also hemp, deserves to be entirely avoided. There is no room for two opinions on this. Some think alcohol may be taken as medicine. However, doctors in Europe, which is the home of wine, say that even this is not necessary. At first alcohol was used there for many ailments, but that has now been stopped. As a matter of fact, this whole argument is advanced with dubious motives. If wine can be used for medicinal purposes [the argument runs], there can be no objection against its use as drink either; that is the game of these advocates of drink. But aloes and crotons are good medicine; yet no one suggests that they be used as food. It is possible that alcohol may prove beneficial in certain illnesses, but the havoc that it has wrought is so great that it is the duty of every thoughtful person to give up even its medicinal use, at the cost of his life if need be. If, by using alcohol for preserving the body, we are likely to harm the best interests of hundreds of people, our duty requires that we sacrifice the body instead. There are in India hundreds of thousands who do not take alcohol in spite of the doctor's orders. They are not willing to prolong their lives by taking alcohol or anything else to which they have an objection. The great people of China, enslaved by opium as they are, will soon perish in spite of the freedom that they have achieved. The *garasias*[2] among us have lost their patrimony, thanks to their addiction to opium.

The reader will easily recognize the harm in alcohol, hemp and opium, but not so readily that in cigarettes and tobacco. These have spread their tentacles so firmly over the human race that it will take ages to free it of them. Young and old, all alike have got into their clutches. Even people regarded as virtuous have taken to smoking and the habit is not regarded as something to be ashamed of. It is quite a popular form of hospitality among friends. Instead of being checked, the habit is spreading. The ordinary man is not even aware of the fact that cigarette dealers use every kind of trick in the manufacture of cigarettes to confirm the hold of the addiction over its victims.

Various kinds of perfumed solutions[3] and even opium water, are sprinkled on the tobacco. As a result of these practices, cigarettes acquire a stronger and stronger hold over us. Thousands of pounds are spent on advertisement in order to popularize them. Cigarette companies in Europe run their own printing presses. They purchase bioscopes and offer all kinds of prizes, start lotteries and spend money like water on advertisements. The result is that even women have begun to smoke. Poems have been written about the cigarette, which has been called the poor man's friend.

It is impossible to estimate the harm done by smoking. A

smoker becomes so brazen-faced that, indifferent to the feelings of others, he will light his cigarette even in another's house without so much as asking for permission to do so. He respects no one's presence.

It has been observed that cigarette or tobacco smokers will commit many other crimes in order to obtain these things. Children steal money from their parents, in gaol, prisoners treasure stolen cigarettes at great risk. They can get on without food but not without cigarettes. During war, soldiers addicted to smoking are in a pitiable condition if they do not get cigarettes. They become practically useless.

The late Tolstoy, writing on this subject, tells the story of a man who planned to kill his beloved. He drew his knife and got ready to use it. Then he relented and turned back. After this, he sat down for a smoke. The fumes of the cigarette entered his head, the poison affected his brain and he finally committed the murder. It was Tolstoy's firm belief that the cigarette is so subtle a form of intoxication that it should be regarded as in some ways a greater menace than even drink.

Smoking is also very expensive and, indeed, every smoker feels the strain of the expense to a greater of lesser degree, depending on his means. Some people spend five pounds or seventy-five rupees a month on cigarettes. The author has himself come across such a case. Smoking weakens the digestion, renders food tasteless so that more and more spices have to be added to it. The smoker's breathe is offensive. The smoke that he exhales pollutes the atmosphere. At times he gets small ulcers in the mouth. Gums and teeth become black or yellow, and some persons have even contracted serious diseases in consequence. It seems strange that people who disapprove of drinking see nothing wrong in smoking; when, however we remember how subtle is the poison of smoking, we see easily enough why it is that men who hate alcohol are nevertheless ready to enjoy smoking. Those who wish to remain healthy should definitely give up the cigarette.

Drink, tobacco, hemp, etc., not damage physical health but also impair mental fitness and entail wasteful expenditure. We lose all our moral sense and become salves to our weakness.

About tea, coffee and cocoa, however, it seems extremely

difficult to explain the truth and convince anyone that they are harmful.

One must say, all the same, that they, too, are harmful. These also contain some kinds of intoxicants. If milk and sugar were not added to tea and coffee, they would have no nutritional value whatever. experiments in living exclusively on tea and coffee indicate that they contain no nourishment for the blood. Only a few years ago, tea and coffee were generally not drunk among us. They were only taken on certain occasions or with medicine, but, tidy in the wake of modern progress, they have become a daily necessity. They are offered even to a casual visitor and frequent tea-parties are given. During Lord Curzon's regime, tea wrought terrible havoc. That gentleman, seeking to promote the interests of tea merchants, introduced tea into every household so that those who were previously accustomed to wholesome drinks now take tea.

Cocoa has not yet become so popular because it is slightly more expensive that tea. Fortunately for us, we have not yet made friends with it, but it holds strong enough sway in fashionable homes.

Tea, coffee and cocoa, all have a certain property that weakens out digestive powers, they are intoxicants because they form a habit which cannot be broken. When the author was in the habit of drinking tea, he felt lethargic if he did not get tea at the usual hour—this is the conclusive test of an intoxicant. On one occasion, about 400 women and children were gathered together at a function. The organizing committee had resolved not to provide tea or coffee. The women in the gathering were in the habit of taking tea at four every afternoon.

A message was soon conveyed to the organizers that, if tea was not served, the ladies would fall ill and be unable to move. And so the resolve had to be set aside. As arrangements were being make for serving tea, excited messages poured in demanding that the organizers should hurry up, The ladies' heads had begun to ache and every moment felt like a month to them. It was only after they had their tea that these worthy ladies' face brightened up and they calmed down.

This incident has been described exactly as it happened. One woman had suffered so much harm because of the tea habit that she could not digest any food and had constant headaches. Her health, however, has greatly improved since she, with a strong effort of will, gave up tea. A physician in the employ of Battersea Municipality in England has discovered that thousands of women in that area suffer from nervous disorders, which he ascribes to their addiction to tea. The author has come upon innumerable examples of the harm done to health by tea and he is personally convince, therefore, that tea is very injurious to health.

As regards coffee, there is a couplet which has become well known:

> Counters phlegm and wind,[4] but lower vigour and strength
> And turns blood to water—two merits against three faults.

This verse sounds quite convincing. Coffee may have the virtue of counteracting phlegm and wind. But so have some other substances. Those who wish to drink coffee for the first two reasons should take a little ginger juice; it will serve the same purpose as coffee. But a preparation detrimental to vigour which needs to be fully conserved, one reducing strength and turning blood into water, surely deserves to be wholly shunned.

Cocoa shares the defects of coffee. Like tea, it also contains a substance which has the effect of making the skin quite rough.

For those who include morals in their conception of good health, there is a further argument against these three beverages. Tea, coffee and cocoa are produced for the most part by indentured labour. In cocoa plantations. Negro workers are subjected to such inhuman treatment that if we witnessed it with our own eyes we would have no desire to drink cocoa. Volumes have been written on the tortures inflicted in these plantations. To be sure, if we made searching inquiries regarding the origin of the various articles of our diet, we should feel called upon to reject 90 per cent of them!

In place of these three drinks, a harmless and nourishing beverage can be prepared in the following manner. Those who like can certainly call it tea. Many coffee lovers cannot distinguish it from coffee. Wheat should be well cleaned and roasted in a pan. It should be kept on the fire till it becomes red and is about to turn black. It should then be taken off the fire and ground rough in a coffee-mill.

A teaspoon of this powder should be put into a cup and boiling water poured over it. Boiling this mixture for a minute improves the flavour.

Milk and sugar to taste may be added but it can also be taken without them. Every reader will find it worthwhile to make this experiment. If he acquires this habit and gives up tea, coffee and cocoa, he will save such money and also be spared the risk to his health. Those who do not want the bother of roasting and grinding the wheat may send 9b. to the Manager, and they will receive one lb, of the prepared wheat powder.

[From Gujarati] *Indian Opinion,* 8-3-1913

NOTES

1. *Vide* "Letter to Secretary for Interior", 15-3-1913.
2. Land-owners inheriting shares of state lands in virtue of relationship with the ruling family.
3. Literally, "acids".
4. The original has *kaph* and *vayu*—terms in Ayurveda, a system of Indian medicine.

11
General Knowledge About Health-XI

We have seen that certain things should be avoided altogether. It remains to be shown that there are others which, for quite different reasons, should either be given up or consumed only in limited quantities. Postponing this discussion for the moment, we shall consider what our diet ought to be.

We can divide mankind into three very large categories on the basis of diet. To one class belong the people who, by choice or necessity, eat vegetable products only. This is the largest class. It consists of most persons in India and Europe and considerable numbers in Japan and China. Of these people, a few are vegetarians as a matter of religious principle, but the majority do without meat because they are unable to obtain it, though, if they get it, they eat it with relish. Among these latter are included Italians, Irish and Scottish people and the poor of Russia as well as of China and Japan. Thus, the chief food of Italy is macaroni, of Ireland potato, of Scotland oatmeal and of China and Japan, rice. People of the second category eat a little meat or fish in addition to vegetable products, once or more than once a day. The majority in England comes under this category, as do rich Muslims in India and Hindus who are unorthodox, besides the well-to-do Chinese and Japanese. This division, though quite large, is very much smaller that the first one. The third division consists of primitive tribes inhabiting the Arctic regions, as well as some Negroes who live on flesh alone. Their number is very small and even these, as they come into contact with European travellers, are learning to add vegetables to their diet. The conclusion to be drawn from all this simply is that man can live in all the three ways; what we have to consider, however, is the question as to which diet is the most health giving.

The structure of the body would seem to indicate that Nature intended man to be a vegetarian. A comparison which other animals reveals that our body structure most closely resembles that of fruit eating animals, that is, the apes. The diet of the apes is fresh and dry fruit. Their teeth and stomach are similar to ours. The teeth and the stomach of predacious beasts, such as the lion and the tiger, differ in structure from ours. We do not have claws as they have. We have, moreover, something in common with non-carnivorous beasts—the ox, for instance. We do not, however, possess intestines like theirs and in the same number, for digesting large quantities of grass. From this, many scientists conclude that man is not by nature carnivorous nor is he formed so as to be able to eat every kind of vegetable food. Even from among vegetable products, fruit alone should be his staple diet.

Chemists have shown by experiment that fruits contain all the elements necessary for the maintenance of human life. Fruits such as bananas, oranges, dates, figs, apples, pineapples, almonds, walnuts, peanuts and coconuts contain all the elements necessary for health and energy. These scientists say that this food need not be cooked, and as animals maintain health by eating sun-ripened fruit, so should we. They go so far as to assert that cooking removes certain essential properties of vegetable foods and reduces their nutritional value. The stimulating quality peculiar to vegetable products is partly lost in the process. They even advance the argument that vegetable products which cannot be eaten raw are no diet for us.

If this argument is correct, surely much of the time spent in preparing and eating food be saved and we could finish our meals in a shorter time. Much of the time of our womenfolk and the space take up by kitchens, etc., in our homes would then be saved and we would be free to attend to many other matters by putting to good use the time and money thus saved.

The idea that all cooking will stop, that women will be set free from the prison-house of the kitchen, that women will themselves desire such freedom—all this will, I am afraid, seem a mere dream and some may ask why at all we should discuss things which are impossible. We are, however, not concerned at the moment with whether everyone can put this into practice. We are only thinking of what is best to do. If we know what is perfect health, we shall achieve a more or less satisfactory level of health. If we know what the ideal diet is, we shall know what we should generally eat.

Many books have been written on this subject in Europe. One even comes across Europeans who experiment with fruit diet. Some of them have recorded their experiences. These men take to a fruit diet not from any religious consideration but purely for the sake of health. There is a German named Just who has written an excellent book[1] in which he has proved, with numerous examples, that fruit diet is the best. He has cured many patients merely with the help of fruit diet and fresh air. He even claims that men can get all the nourishment they need from the fruit growing in their own regions.

It will not be out of place if I here describe my own experiment. For the past six months, I have eaten nothing but fruits. I have not taken even milk or curds. My diet has consisted of bananas, peanuts, olive oil, lemon or similar citrus fruit, and dates. I do not claim that the experiment has proved completely successful. Six months is not enough to gauge the results of such a big change, but I can say this at any rate, that when others fell ill I remained well. I have greater physical and mental energy, than before. As regards physical strength, I may not be able, I admit, to lift as heavy weights as I could formerly, but I can work for longer periods at a stretch without fatigue. Of mental work I do much more at present and cope with it all. I have recommended this diet to some patients and the results have been little short of miraculous. I intend to describe these in the chapter on diseases. In fine, then, the experience of others and of myself and what reading and thinking I have done seem to suggest that a fruit diet is superior to all other kinds of diet.

I do not for a moment expect that anyone reading this will straightaway take to experimenting with fruit diet. What I have will scarcely have any effect on the reader. But, if I am to tell the truth, as I wish to, I think it is my duty to present only my own conclusions, such as they are.

If, however, any reader does plan to experiment with fruit diet. I would advise him not to rush into it but to go slow. After first reading all the chapters, he should draw his own conclusions and then do whatever he wants to with full deliberation.

In the following section we shall consider the diet of the second category. I think the conclusions of that section will be more acceptable and also that, after he has perused it, he will find it easier to understand the present section.

To those who have been following these chapters seriously, my request is that they form their own opinions and that, too, after reading the entire series.

[From Gujarati] *Indian Opinion,* 15-3-1913

NOTE

1. Return to Nature.

12
General Knowledge About Health-XII

On the next level and below fruits, comes vegetable diet. This consists of all kinds of vegetables, cereals, pulses, beans, milk, etc. Just as fruit-diet contains all the elements that man needs, so too does vegetarian diet, though the two do not have the same effect. Some of the elements we obtain from food are also to be found in the air; yet we cannot obtain them from air and do without food. Moreover, all vegetable products lose something of their original nature when cooked and are to that extent robbed of value, one would have cooked food and cannot go without vegetables, it has to be considered what it would be best to take.

Among grains, wheat is the best. Man can live on wheat alone. It contains all the nutritive elements in good proportion. Many preparations can be made of it, and it is also easy to digest. Children's foods available in the market also contain a proportion of wheat. In the same category with wheat are millets and maize, from all of the which *rotli*[1] or *roti*[2] can be prepared, though these cereals cannot compare with wheat. It is important to understand what the best way of taking wheat is. Wheat flour, which we know as mill-flour, is absolutely worthless, devoid of all nutritional value. Dr. Alinson says that a dog he kept exclusively on such a diet succumbed as a result, but another flourished on bread from a different variety of flour.

White flour is entirely devoid of bran, which is the source of the taste and energy-giving property of wheat. White bread is in such demand because, eaten with it, other tasty things are most enjoyed. For instance, those who eat cheese derive energy from it but they eat it, and can eat it, only as an adjunct to bread. *Rotli*, too made of such flour is bad; it is tough and offers neither taste not nutrition. *The best flour is that which is obtained by grinding clean wheat at home* and if in addition, it is ground by hand in a quern, it is considered to be the very best. If, however, one cannot secure a quern, one can purchase at a low cost a hand mill to be kept in the home and grind wheat for personal use. Or one can buy un sifted Boer-meal and use it. The flour should be used as it is, un sifted, The *roti* made of this flour is tasty and nourishing and the flour is more economical to use than *maida*, since, being nutritious, it cannot be consumed in the same quantity as *maida*.

It should be borne in mind that ready-made bread is quite worthless. Whether white or brown, it is adulterated. Moreover, it is prepared from flour fermented with yeast. This is a great drawback. It is the opinion of many experienced people that bread made of such flour is harmful. Then again, during preparation, the loaf is covered with *tandul* or fat; hence, it should be unacceptable both to Hindus and Muslims. *To eat shop bread in place of roti prepared at home is nothing but a mark of laziness.*

Another easy and pleasant way of eating wheat is to grind it coarse and make porridge from it. Porridge, if well cooked in water and taken with milk or sugar, tastes delicious and is much superior to other kinds of food.

Rice seems to contain no nutriment and it is doubtful whether man could live on it alone, unless pulses, ghee and milk are added to it. Wheat, on the other hand, cooked in water alone is enough to maintain one in good health.

Vegetables are eaten mainly for their taste. They have a laxative effect and thus help purify the blood. However, they are of the nature of grass, they are difficult to digest and give excessive work to the stomach. Everyone must have noticed that those who are given to consuming vegetables in excessive quantities are of the delicate constitution and are called *pepchidas*[3]. They frequently suffer from dyspepsia and are always swallowing medicines for indigestion. That some varieties of vegetables are a form of grass is plain enough to us.

Vegetables, therefore, should certainly be eaten but, be it remembered, only in small quantities.

Pulses—beans, *val*,[4] *tuwar*,[5] vetches, tare, lentil—are regarded as good tonic foods. They are difficult to digest as they require much heat in the stomach. The fact that a person who has eaten a quantity of pulses frequently passes wind only means that he has not been able to carry it. It is for this reason that pulses are regarded as causing *vayu* [excess of wind]. One characteristic of pulses is that they keep one going for a fairly long time. A person who has to undertake much physical labour can tolerate pulses more easily and even derive some benefit from them. We, however, who do limited physical work generally cannot afford to eat an excess of pulses. Those who loll in cushioned seats cannot eat the same type or quantity of food as labourers.

A famous writer in England named Dr. Haig has proved with numerous experiments that pulses are a very unwholesome food.

They produce an excess of a particular acid in the body which causes many ailments and brings on premature old age. He has given many reasons to explain why this happens, which there is no need to consider here. My personal experience, at any rate, indicates that it is harmful to eat pulses. Those, however, who cannot master their palate may eat them, but with care.

[From Gujarati] *Indian Opinion,* 22-3-1913

NOTES

1. Unleavened bread.
2. *Ibid.*
3. Gujarati colloquial expression meaning "milksop".
4. Varieties of pulses.
5. *Ibid.*

13
General Knowledge About Health-XIII

We shall now consider what vegetables should be avoided. In almost every part of India, it is customary to use chillies together with spices such as coriander seed, black pepper, etc. The practice does not obtain in other parts of the world to the same extent. If we offer any of our spicy dishes to the Negroes here, they also will hesitate to eat them as they do not care for their taste. Many white who are unused to spices are totally unable to eat our pungent food and, if they force themselves to eat it, their digestion suffers and the mouth gets inflamed. I have witnessed this myself in the case of some whites. We may conclude, therefore, that spices are not themselves appetizing but that, having become accustomed to them by long use, we like their smell and taste. We have already recognized, however, that eating anything for the sake of its taste is harmful to health.

Let us then examine why people eat spices. They do so, it will be readily admitted, in order to be able to eat more and digest more.

Chillies, coriander seed, cummin, etc., produce heat in the stomach and in consequence we seem to feel more hungry. If, however, we imagine from this that the food we have thus consumed is all digested and transformed into pure blood, we shall be sadly mistaken. Many people indulge in over-spicy food. Their stomachs become very weak in the long-run and some even get attacks of sprue. A certain man used to eat large amounts of chillies, a habit which he could not overcome, and he died in his youth after a long illness which kept him on bed for six months. It is imperative that we eliminate spices from out diet altogether.

This stricture applies equally to salt. No one will like this idea and some may even be aghast at it, but its truth has, nevertheless, been proved by experience. An association has been started in England whose creed is that salt is even more injurious than most spices. Our diet supplies salt to us in organic forms, and that is all that we really need. Sea-salt and rock-salt, on the other hand, are superfluous and when consumed are expelled again through perspiration and otherwise. This means that salt has no specific utility for the body. One book goes so far as to say that consumption of salt has a toxic effect on the blood and that one who has abstained from salt for many years and has otherwise kept his body clean has his blood stream so pure that even snake-bite will do him no harm; for the blood of such a person develops a resistance to the venom. We cannot ascertain the truth of this statement but from experience I can at least say that ailments such as cough, piles, asthma, bleeding, etc., respond immediately to a saltless diet. A certain Indian had long suffered from asthma and cough. These were cured by the adoption of a saltless diet together with the use of the usual remedies. I have not come across any undesirable results from giving up salt. I myself gave it up over two years ago and have felt no ill effect; on the contrary, I observe some beneficial effects. I need less water and feel less lethargic. The incident which occasioned my giving up salt was somewhat unusual, too. The person[1] whose ailment was responsible for my doing so has had her illness under control ever since. I am confident, too, that had the patient been able to give salt completely, her malady would have been entirely eradicated. I have observed during numerous experiments that people find it difficult to give up green vegetables and pulses together with the salt but this has to be done. I think these articles prove hard to digest without the addition of salt. This does not mean that salt stimulates digestion; on the contrary, just as chillies merely give the illusion of aiding the digestive process and are found to be harmful in the long run, so it is with salt. It follows, therefore, that those who adopt a saltless diet must give up green vegetables and pulses as well. Anyone can make this experiment and watch the effect on himself. Just as an opium addict who tries to rid himself of his habit feels out of sorts and weak at first, so is the case with one who refrains from salt. One should not, however, lose heart on this account. If the person who gives up salt is patient enough, he will be rewarded by and by.

The writer has been bold enough to assert that even milk is among the articles to be avoided. One basis for this opinion is his own experience, but that should be kept out of consideration. We entertain so strong a superstition as to the value of milk that it would be a vain effort to combat it. The writer does not expect that his readers will agree with all the opinions he expresses in these articles, nor does he expect either that all those who approve of them will put them into practice; his object is only to present his ideas, leaving it to others to accept whatever they will. There is nothing wrong, therefore, in his writing even about milk. Many doctors have stated that milk is the cause of typhoid. Pamphlets have been published on this subject. Milk gets easily contaminated with airborne germs and those which are inimical to health multiply rapidly in it. We have to take a great deal of trouble to keep it in good condition. In South Africa there are special laws for [the protection of] consumers of milk. Very many recommendation are made for the preservation and storage of milk and cleaning of utensils. It seems reasonable to question whether it is worth while using an article which needs so much care to keep and which, if not so guarded, may do harm.

Moreover, the goodness or otherwise of milk depends on the condition of the cow and what she eats. Doctors cite instances of persons drinking the milk of a tuberculous cow and themselves developing tuberculosis. It is difficult to find a perfectly healthy cow, and the milk of a diseased cow is unwholesome. It is well known that a sick mother's milk makes the baby also sick. When a baby which has not yet been weaned falls ill, *vaids* treat the mother, so that through her milk the medicine may act on the baby. What is true of woman's milk applies also to cow's milk. In this way, the food and the health of the giver of milk have an intimate bearing on its consumer. Would not the right course be to avoid this milk, the consumption of which demands so much trouble and carries so much risk? The strength giving property of milk is to be found in other substance as well.

Olive oil is a good substitute for milk in many ways. A preparation of sweet almonds made by soaking them in hot water, peeling and grinding them to a fine paste and mixing this thoroughly with water, will have all the beneficial properties of milk and none of its risks.

Finally, let us consider the law of Nature: a calf gives up sucking after a few months and, as soon as its teeth are developed, it turns to food which requires their use; this should be the rule with human beings, too. We are meant to take milk only so long as we are infants. We, too, should, when our teeth are grown, employ them in chewing fresh fruit such as apples and dry fruit such as almonds, or *rotli*. This is not the place to calculate how much money and time can be saved by anyone who has shaken off his slavery to milk, but each one will be able to find out for himself. Milk-products, too, are unnecessary. The acid content of why is available from lemon and its other nutrients from almonds, etc. As to ghee, thousands of Indians consume oil instead.

Let us now turn for a while to the third type of diet. It is a mixture of vegetarian and non-vegetarian elements. This diet is adopted by a large number of people, of whom many suffer from various ailments and many others are found to be healthy. That we are not meant to be meat-eaters, each one of our organs and the constitution of our bodies make evident. Dr. Kingsford and Dr. Haig have vividly described the ill effects of non-vegetarian diet on the body. They have proved that the acid produced by consumption of pulses is also produced by that of meat. Meat-eating damages the teeth and causes rheumatism. It makes a man more prone to anger, and therefore, a sick man. According to our definition of health, one who is quick to get angry cannot be counted a healthy person.

Those who eat the fourth and last type of diet, that is, who subsist exclusively on flesh, need not detain us here. Their state is so vile that the very thought of them should be enough to put us off meat-eating. They are not healthy in any sense of the term. As soon as they come up a little and get some knowledge, they tend to accept a vegetarian diet.

What all this adds up to is that very few people will be found ready for an exclusively fruit diet, but that a diet of dry and fresh fruit, wheat and olive oil is worth a trial, it being possible to maintain sound health on it. Among fruits, bananas occupy the first place.

Besides, dates, plums and figs are strength-giving fruits. Fresh grapes improve the blood. Orange, lemons and apples can be mixed with bananas and eaten with *rotlis*. The addition of olive oil to *rotli* does not impair its taste. Such a diet costs very little trouble or money and does not require salt and chillies, milk or sugar. Plain sugar is an absolutely useless article of food. People who are very fond of sweets lose their teeth early and the sweet food does them no good in any way. Wheat, almonds, peanuts, walnuts, fresh fruits—from every on of these a number of edible preparations can be made.

What we have now to consider is how much food to eat and when; this we shall do in the next chapter.

[From Gujarati] *Indian Opinion*, 29-3-1913

NOTE

1. Kasturba Gandhi.

14
General Knowledge About Health-XIV[1]

6. HOW MUCH AND HOW OFTEN TO EAT

We have considered what the ideal diet should be. It is necessary to inquire how much and how often to eat, and the topic calls for a separate article. To some extent the two questions, "How much should one eat?" and "How often should one eat?" are interrelated. I say "to some extent" because one cannot, and one should not, eat at a single meal the total quantity of food to be consumed in one day, so that "how much to eat" and "how often" are not so closely interrelated.

Doctors differ widely on the question: how much one should eat. "In plenty", says one doctor, and he recommends different amounts of various foods according to their properties. Another in August-December 1942, during his incarceration in the Agakhan Palace at Poona, Gandhiji wrote in Gujarati what became, in its English translation by Dr. Sushila Nayyar, *Key to Health*, published by Navajivan Publishing House, Ahmedabad, in 1948. While this book was not based on the series of articles published in *Indian Opinion*, according to Gandhiji, it did not fundamentally differ from them. Doctor says that physical and mental workers should eat different kinds and quantities of food. A third opines that a labourer and a prince should eat the same quantity of food—that it is simply not true that a prince can make do with less but a labourer must have more.

Everyone knows that a weak man and a strong man need different quantities of food. The diet of a man differs from that of a woman.

There is a difference in the quantities of food for adults and children, for the aged and the young. Lastly, there is one writer who even states that, if the food is so thoroughly masticated that it turns into liquid and is swallowed with ease like saliva, we would find two to four ounces of food quite sufficient. He has carried out thousands of experiments. His book has been sold by the thousand and is widely read. Such being the position, it is useless to recommend definite quantities of food; most doctors have said, however, that 99 per cent eat more than they require. Even otherwise, the thing is simple enough to be obvious to us all. This being so, it is not necessary to prescribe a minimum diet for fear that people might eat loo little. To tell the truth, what needs to be emphasized is that, while planning a diet, all of us should cut down on the quantity we consume.

As mentioned above, food should be thoroughly masticated. By this means, we shall be able to extract the utmost nourishment from even a small quantity of food and gain in every way. It has been shown that the faces of one who eats only as much as he can comfortably digest are small, well formed, darkish, sticky, dry and free from bad odour. One whose faeces are not so formed must have eaten excessive and unsuitable food and failed to masticate it and mix it with the saliva in his mouth. Thus, from the appearance of our faeces we can make out if we have eaten too much. He whose tongue is coated on rising, who sleeps uneasily and dreams frequently, must have been eating too much. One who has to get up often at night to pass urine must have taken too much liquid. By such detailed observation, anyone can decide the quantity of food required by him. Many people have offensive breath. Clearly, they have not digested their food. At times, those who over-eat get boils and pimples on the face and in the nostrils. But we do not take these affections seriously. Some get continuous hiccups. Others suffer from flatulence. *The simple meaning of all these ailments is that we have turned our stomach into a commode and that we carry this commode with us wherever we go.*

If we could spare the time to think quietly about this matter, we would thoroughly despise our own habits. We would definitely eat less and put an end to dinners and feasts, would make it a rule never to attend or give community dinners. Our hospitality would take an altogether different form, much to our own relief and that of the guest. As for dinner parties, one would forget the very mention of them. We do not invite people to join us when we clean our teeth or when we drink water. Eating a meal is a similar bodily function. Why do we go fussing all over in performing it? Every time we have a guest, we must not make things unbearable both for him and us. The explanation is that our palate has been spoilt through constant indulgence, so that we trump up one excuse after another for eating something. We feed our guest sumptuously in the hope of being similarly treated at his house.

Actually, we seek such occasions so that we can have more opportunities of feasting on rich dishes. If we asked someone with a wholesome body to smell our mouth about an hour after we have indulged in such eating and heard his comments, we would certainly have cause to be ashamed of ourselves. There are even some young gourmets who, in order to be able to enjoy eating, take fruit salt immediately after a meal or vomit out what they have already consumed and then fall to eating the sweets again.

To a greater or lesser extent, we all behave like this. That is why our great men laid down for us certain religious observances like fasts, *rozas*[2], etc. There are numerous fast days among Roman Catholics too.

There is nothing wrong whatever in anyone fasting completely or partially once in a fortnight purely for the sake of good health. It will do him a world of good indeed. The practice followed by many Hindus of eating only once a day during the *chaturmas*[3] is based on considerations of health. When the air is humid and the day is overcast most of the time, the digestion becomes slack and one should, therefore, eat less at such times.

Let us now consider how often one should eat. Most people in India eat only twice a day. Those who eat thrice will be found to belong to the labouring classes. People learnt eating four times only when they began to ape English ways. Recently, certain societies have been formed in England and America. Their function is to persuade the public to refrain from taking more than two meals a day. They has no need to eat either much or often.

[From Gujarati] *Indian Opinion,* 5-4-1913

NOTES

1. Articles in this series were later published as a book which was translated into Hindi and other Indian languages. Based on the Hindi version was *A Guide to Health*, an English adaptation by A. Rama Iyer, published by S. Ganesan, Madras, in July 1921. The book was translated into several European languages.
2. Fasts observed by Muslims from sunrise to sunset, during the month of *Ramzan*.
3. The four monsoon months, from about mid-July to mid-November, during which pious Hindus observe partial fasts advise us to go without breakfast. The night's sleep serves the purpose of food. At daybreak, therefore, we are ready not for food but for work. They believe that we are ready for food only after two or three hours of work. These men, therefore, eat only twice a day and do not even drink tea, etc., between meals. A well-known doctor called Dewey has written a book on this subject in which he has described in a convincing manner the benefits accruing from fasting, cutting out breakfast, generally eating less, etc. My own experience during the past eight years is that, after the period of youth is past, there is absolutely no need for anyone to eat more than twice a day. Once a person's body is fully grown and further development has stopped.

15
General Knowledge About Health-XV

7. EXERCISE

Exercise is just as essential to mankind as are air, water and food, though it is true that man cannot get on for a long time without air, water and food as he can without exercise. It is a fact of common experience, however, that one cannot enjoy really good health without exercise. We have to interpret exercise in the same way that we did "food". Exercise does not necessarily mean *moidanda*[1], football, cricket or going out for a walk. Exercise means physical and mental activity. Just as food is necessary for the mind as much as for bones and flesh, so also is exercise necessary both for body and mind. If the body has no exercise, it is sickly and, if the mind has none, it is dull.

Stupidity should also be regarded only as a kind of illness. It betrays sheer ignorance to describe as healthy a wrestler who, though adept at wrestling, is mentally a boor. There is a saying in English that he alone is healthy who has a sound mind in a sound body.

What is this exercise? Nature has so arranged things for us that we can be continuously taking exercise in one way or another. If we but think calmly enough, we shall see that a majority of people in the world live on agriculture. All members in a farmer's family have some form of exercise. It is only if they work eight, ten or even more hours every day in the fields or elsewhere that they can get their daily bread. They need no separate exercise for the mind. A farmer cannot work without applying his mind. He must be able to test the nature of his soil, must watch changes of weather, must know how to manipulate his plough skilfully and be generally familiar with the movements of the stars, the sun and the moon. However, clever a city-dweller may be, every time he goes to a farmer's house, he feels altogether out of his element. The farmer can say how seed should be sown; he is familiar with all the by-ways in the vicinity and knows all the men in the neighbourhood. By looking at the stars he can judge the direction even at night. He can make certain deductions from the voice and speed of birds; for instance, when certain birds cluster or sing together, he sees in it a sign of the approach of the monsoon or some other similar phenomenon. Thus, the farmer knows enough of astronomy, geography and geology to serve his needs. He has to feed his children and has, therefore, some idea of the duties of man, and, residing as he does in the vast open spaces of this earth, he naturally becomes aware of the greatness of God. Physically, it goes without saying, he is always sturdy. He is his own physician, when ill. Thus, we can see, he does have an educated mind.

But all men are not going to be farmers. Moreover, these chapters are not being written for the benefit of farmers. The question is, what should those who have gone into business or some similar profession do in this regard? The farmer's life has been described at some length in order that we may find a rational answer to this problem, that we who are not farmers can arrange our way of life somewhat on the pattern of his and that we may realize that, in so far as our manner of living differs from the farmer's, we would enjoy poorer health. We can conclude from a farmer's way of living that a man should do physical work for eight hours a day and that of a kind that would stimulate our mental powers in the very process of doing it.

Now, merchants and others certainly obtain mental exercise in the course of their work, but this is one-sided. A business man does not know astronomy or geography or history, as the farmer does. He may be able to judge about movements of prices and may be proficient in the art of salesmanship, but this is not enough to exercise fully his mental faculties. In this type of work, the body does perform some movements now and then, but they are too slight to be of any account.

In the West, they have invented games like cricket for such people. Another way is to observe some days in the year as holidays, when more games are played, and to do some light reading by way of mental exercise. This is one method which we may consider. To be sure, spending time in sports does give some exercise to the body, but exercise of this kind does nothing to improve the mind. We can see the truth of this from numerous instances. What proportion of men of high intellectual calibre shall we find among those who regularly play cricket or from among the large number who play football? In India, what do we observe as regards the mental development of the princes who give their time to sports? Again, how many of those with well-developed intellectual powers are sportsmen? Experience shows that highly intellectual men are seldom sportsmen as well. The British nowadays are very much given to sports. Their own poet, Kipling, has described these sportsmen as enemies of the mind, and adds that they will also prove themselves enemies to their country. In India, our intellectuals seem to have found a different way. They provide exercise for their minds but relatively very little or none for their bodies.

These people are lost to us. Their bodies are enfeebled by excessive intellectual work. They are continually pursued by some ailment or other and just when they have gained enough experience to be of real use to the country, they pass away. From this we may conclude that neither exercising the brain alone nor the body alone is enough and also that exercise which serves no useful purpose, namely, that derived from sports, has little meaning. Real exercise is that which trains, continuously, both mind and body alike. He alone who takes such exercise can preserve good health. The farmer is the only such person.

Then, what are those to do who are not farmers? The exercise obtained from sports such as cricket leaves much to be desired. We must, therefore, think of a form of exercise something like what the farmer gets. Businessmen and others similarly placed can make a garden round their house and regularly spend two to four hours a day digging there. Hawkers get exercise from their own work itself. If we are living in a rented room, we should not raise any difficulty about working in another's land, for that would indicate a small mind. We would derive nothing but benefit from working on land, whosoever's it might be. The appearance of our house would be improved and we would have the satisfaction of having looked after another's land. It is necessary to say a few words for those who cannot find an opportunity to work on land or who do not favour such work in any circumstances.

Apart from working on land, the best form of exercise is walking. It has been truly described as the king of physical exercises.

Our *fakirs* and *sadhus* are very healthy. One reason for this is that they do not use horses, carriages or other vehicles. Their journeys are always performed on foot. There has been a famous American writer named Thoreau[2], who has written a highly thought-provoking book on the subject of walking. According to him, the writings of one who refuses to leave his house on the excuse of lack of time and who undertakes no physical activity, are bound to be anaemic like himself. Speaking of his own experience, he says that when he wrote his best books he was doing his longest walking. He thought nothing of walking four or five hours at a stretch. Just as we cannot work when we are hungry, so it should be with exercise. We do not know how to measure mental work, therefore, we arc not able to realize that mental work done unaccompanied by physical exercise will inevitably be dull and ineffectual. Walking results in rapid circulation of blood in all the parts of the body, promotes movements in every organ and strengthens it. One should remember that the arms move during walking.

We obtain fresh air by going for a walk and behold the beauties of Nature. One should not take walks always in the same place or in narrow lanes but go out into fields and groves. We will then be able to appreciate in some measure the beauty of Nature. A walk of a mile or two can scarcely be called walking. A walk, to be worth the name, should cover ten or twelve miles. Those who cannot do this regularly can take long walks on Sundays. A certain patient, who used to suffer from indigestion, went one day to an experienced *vaidya*[3] for some pills. The *vaidya* advised him to take short but regular walks. The patient protested that he was too weak. The *vaidya* realized that he was, in fact, a timid man. He thereupon took the patient with him in his carriage. On the way he purposely dropped his whip. The patient, out of politeness, had to get out to pick it up. The *vaidya* immediately drove off. The poor patient had to follow, panting hard for breath.

The *vaidya* having made sure that the former had covered a fairly long distance, turned the carriage back, picked him up and told him that, since walking was the only medicine for him, he—the *vaidya*—had forced him to walk even at the risk of appearing cruel.

By this time, however, the patient was ravenously hungry and had forgotten all about the whip episode. He thanked the doctor, went home and ate his fill. Those who are not in the habit of walking and suffer from indigestion and its accompanying ills should try the experiment.

[From Gujarati] *Indian Opinion,* 12-4-1913

NOTES

1. An Indian game.
2. Henry David Thoreau (1817-62); American philosopher, naturalist and writer; author, among others, of *Walden, or Life in the Woods and Excursions. Vide* also "On the Duty of Civil Disobedience", 7-9-1907.
3. Physician practising *Ayurveda*, an indigenous system of medicine.

16
General Knowledge About Health-XVI

8. ATTIRE

If health depends on diet, it is also affected to some extent by dress. White women, for the sake of what they fancy to be beauty, dress so that their waist and feet should look narrow and fall victims to various ailments in consequence. In China, women's feet are kept so small that even our children's feet are larger in comparison. The practice does great harm to the health of Chinese women. The reader will easily see from these two illustrations that what we wear does, in some measure, affect our health. The choice of our costumes is not, however, in our own hands. We dress the way our elders did and this seems the right thing to do in our present circumstances. The real function of clothes has gone out of people's minds and these have come to serve as symbols of our religion, country, community, etc.

Again, the costumes worn by the labourer and the office-worker differ greatly from each other. It is indeed difficult in these conditions to consider clothes from the point of view of health; it will be useful, though, to give this matter some thought.

The term attire should here be understood to include also shoes, ornaments, etc.

Let us first examine the basic purpose of clothes. In the natural state man wears no clothes. Men and women cover only their private parts, the rest of the body remaining bare. This makes their skin tough and strong. Such men and women find it easy to withstand the rigours of the open air. They do not suddenly catch cold. In the chapter on air, we saw that we breathe not only through the nose but also through the countless pores of the skin. By covering ourselves with clothes, we obstruct this most important function of the skin. In cold countries, man had to cover himself with more and more clothes as he grew more and more lazy. He could no longer bear the cold. In course of time, this became a regular custom. By and by, people came to look upon clothes as a mode of personal adornment, and, ultimately, costumes came to be a means of identifying one's community, etc.

In fact, Nature has provided man with the best dress in his skin.

It is altogether wrong to think that the nude body is ugly. The finest pictures we see are of the naked body. By covering up the normal organs of the body, do we not, as it were, suggest that Nature has made a mistake? The richer we are, the more stylish grows our dress. People dress themselves in a variety of ways and, looking into the mirror, smile with pleasure and congratulate themselves on their appearance.

If custom had not perverted our outlook, we would easily realize that man appeared at his best and enjoyed the finest health in his naked state. The moment he puts on a mere shirt, he detracts by so much from his appearance. As if this were not enough, both men and women *wear jewellery*. There are quite a few men who fetter their legs [with anklets] and put rings on ears and fingers. All these things are dust-traps. *Heaven alone knows what charm there is in them*. As for women, they have broken all bounds. Anklets so heavy that they can scarcely lift their feet, numerous rings in the ears, large rings again in the nose, and no end of bangles on the wrists. By wearing these, we collect a great deal of dirt on the body. The filth in the ears and nose is beyond description. We regard this filthy condition as an ornament and feel constrained to spend money on it. The women do not mind risking their lives at the hands of robbers. It has been truly said that for the folly of pride we pay an unlimited price by way of suffering. Women have refused to have their ear-rings removed, though they have boils in their ears. A bangle cannot be removed, even if there is a boil on the hand and even if the latter has become septic. Be it a he or a she, it would be impairing one's appearance to take off one's diamond ring even when the finger has grown septic! Most people must have personally come across such instances.

It will be difficult to bring about a radical improvement in dress, but we can discard ornaments. We can dispense with garments which do not seem necessary, retain a few in deference to custom and discard the rest. Anyone whose mind has outgrown the fallacious notion that "apparel maketh a man" will be able to effect considerable improvement [in his dress] and safeguard his health.

Now-a-days, moreover, a notion is in the air that it is best for us to put on European dress, that it is more impressive and wins us greater respect from people. This is not the place for a discussion of the topic.

All that needs to be said here is that, though the European costume is suitable for the cold countries of Europe, the Indian costume suits both Hindus and Muslims in India. Our clothes are loose and, therefore, allow free circulation of air. Being white, they disperse the rays of the sun. In dark clothes one feels hotter in the sun because the rays falling on them are not so dispersed,

We always cover our heads, particularly when going out. The turban has become our especial mark declaring us to be Indians.

There will be nothing but benefit, however, from leaving the head uncovered wherever possible. Wearing long hair and parting it with ever so much care seems to be rather uncouth. Dust, dirt, and lice collect in long hair. One will also find it difficult to treat any boils that may develop on one's scalp. For a turban-wearer to grow long hair like a Saheb is sheer absurdity.

We fall into the clutches of many diseases through our feet. The feet of those who wear shoes, etc., become tender. With shoes on, the feet perspire and emit an offensive odour. Anyone sensitive to smell can scarcely bear to stand near such a person when he is removing his shoes and socks, so offensive is the odour of the feet. We call shoes "shields against thorns" or "protectors of the feet", which means that we need wear shoes only when we have to walk among thorns or stir out in extreme heat or cold, and even then, we need cover, not the entire feet, but only the soles; when necessary, therefore, one may put on only sandals. Anyone who suffers from headaches, physical weakness, aching feet, and anyone used to wearing of shoes should try walking barefoot. He will soon discover the advantages of keeping one's feet uncovered, in contact with the earth and free from perspiration.

Sandals are an excellent form of footwear and also comparatively cheap. In Africa, they are made by Trappists[1] near Pinetown for anyone who wants them and one can also get them made in Phoenix.

The average individual will not have the courage to use *sandals* only.

Even such a person should always keep his feet uncovered whenever possible and use *sandals* when he must cover the soles and can do without shoes.

[From Gujarati] *Indian Opinion,* 19-4-1913

NOTE

1. Monks of Cistercian order noted for silence and other austerities.

17
General Knowledge About Health-XVII

9. AN INTIMATE CHAPTER

Those who have carefully followed the chapters on health so far should read this, I submit, with especial care and ponder well over it.

Other chapters are still to follow and will, I feel, prove useful, but there will be none in the series as important as the present one. As I indicated earlier I have in these chapters said nothing on which I have had no personal experience or of which I was not firmly convinced.

There are many things which promote good health, all of them necessary, but the most important is *brahmacharya*[1]. We can have good health by means of good air, water and food; but, if we spend all that we earn, we shall be left with nothing on hand. Similarly, if we fritter away the health which we gain, what remains of our capital behind? For both men and women, therefore, *brahmacharya* is an absolute necessity if they are to preserve the wealth of physical well-being; no one need doubt this. He who has conserved his generative fluid is known as *viryavan*, a man of strength.

What is *brahmacharya*?—it may be asked. It consists in men and women refraining from carnal enjoyment. "Refraining from carnal enjoyment" does not mean merely refraining from contact with each other with such enjoyment in view, but also keeping the mind free from the very thought of it—one must not even dream about it. Man should not be disturbed by the presence of woman and woman by the presence of man. We should hold back and store within our bodies the mysterious power that Nature has bestowed upon us and use it to promote our health, the health not only of the body but also of the mind, the intellect and the memory.

Let us now take a look—at the strange things that go on around us. Most men and women, whether young or old, are submerged in this infatuation. On such occasions we go utterly mad. Our reason ceases to function, a veil seems to come over our eyes and we are blinded with passion. I have observed men, women and young people of both sexes looking distraught when possessed by passion. My personal experience is no different. Whenever, I have been overcome by this state, I have lost all sense. Such is the nature of passion. Thus, for the sake of a grain of pleasure[2], we lose a maund of vitality. When our excitement dies down, we find ourselves in a pitiable state. The following morning our body is heavy, we are ill at ease, and a lethargy sets in. Our mind is out of sorts. In order to set these things right again, or keep them right, we must needs drink milk boiled with spices, swallow iron, take *yakutis*[3], approach *vaidyas* for strength-giving drugs and look around for foods that will serve as aphrodisiacs. Thus, as the days and years go by, we decline in body and mind and find our intellect gone in old age.

This, surely, should not be—in old age, the intellect should grow sharper rather than duller. We should be in such condition that the experience gained during a life-time can be of use to us and to others, a condition possible to those who observe *brahmacharya*. Such a person is unafraid of death and does not forget God even at the moment of death. He does not indulge in vain attempts and does not.

We do not, as a rule, stop to consider that the basic cause of pleasure-hunting, envy, ostentation, hypocrisy, anger, impatience, violent hatred and such other evils is our violation of *brahmacharya*.

If one's mind is not under one's control and one behaves more foolishly even than a child, indulging oneself once every day or oftener, what other crimes would not one commit, knowingly or unknowingly? What unforgivable sins would one stop short of?

But does one ever find anyone observing such *brahmacharya*?

If everyone did so, the world would come to an end. [So

runs the argument.] This is likely to involve a discussion of religious issues. I shall, therefore, pass over that aspect of the matter and consider it from a worldly point of view. In my opinion, both these questions have their origin in our fear and weakness. We do not want to observe *brahmacharya* and, therefore, seek excuses to escape from it. There do exist people, and in large numbers, who observe it; if, however, they were easy to discover, what would be their worth? Thousands of labourers are imprisoned in the bowels of the earth in order that diamonds might be obtained and, even then, only a handful of these are found in a mountain of broken earth and rock. What efforts, then, would be necessary to discover the jewels among men who observe *brahmacharya*? Let us do a simple sum in the rule of three to calculate. If the world comes to an end because we observe *brahmacharya*, how is that any concern of ours? We are not God. He who has created the world will look after His affairs. Whether others observe it or not is not a question for us to ask. When we select business or law or anything else as a career, we do not ask what would happen if everyone became a lawyer or businessman. Finally, those men and women who observe *brahmacharya* will, in the course of time, receive answers to both the questions, that is, they will find others like themselves. And it will also be as plain as daylight to them what will happen to the world if all did the same.

How can these ideas be put into practice by men caught up in worldly responsibilities? What should the married ones do? And those who have children? What should they do who cannot control their desire? We have seen what the ideal is. If we always hold it before us, we shall either be able to follow it faithfully or approximate to it in some measure. If we place before a child the finest models when teaching it to write the letters of the alphabet, it will copy them to the best of its ability. Similarly, we can place before us the ideal of unbroken *brahmacharya*, and then make every effort to approximate to it. What if we happen to be married? The natural law is that men and women should depart from *brahmacharya* only when they desire progeny. If a couple do so after full deliberation, once in a few years, they will not wholly forget themselves and will remain well stored with vitality. Rarely do we come across couples who indulge in sexual intercourse only for the purpose of procreation. The rest in their thousands seek the pleasures of lust, yearn for them and indulge in them. The consequence is that, against their wish, children are born to them. In enjoying these pleasures, we become so utterly blind that we have no consideration for our partner. In this matter men are more guilty than women. In his stupidity man gives no thought to the woman's weakness; he does not stop to consider whether she is strong enough for the burden of bearing children and bringing them up.

People of the West have broken all bounds in this matter. They adopt various techniques so that they may have their pleasure without being burdened with children. Books have been written on these techniques and there are professionals who explain how to indulge in the pleasures of lust and yet have no children! So far at least we have been free from this sin; but we do not think for a moment before imposing burdens on our women and we do not care if our children are weak, lacking in vitality, timid and dull of intellect. Whenever, a child is born, we offer thanks to God. This is only a way of covering up our pitiable condition. *Why should we not regard it a sign of divine anger that we have weak, crippled, lustful and worthless children born to us? What reason for satisfaction can there be over a child of twelve having issues? Why should this be an occasion for merry-making? Why should we not regard it as a manifestation of divine wrath that a girl of twelve should become a mother*? We know that, if a tree bears fruit too soon after it has been planted, the latter is immature and we take good care to see that fruit does not appear too early on a tree. When, on the contrary, we have a celebration on the birth of a child to a child-wife by a child-husband, surely we behave with incredible blindness. Of what good is it to India or the world to be swarmed over with worthless creatures, as with ants? Animals are better off than we are inasmuch as the male and the female are brought together only when we intend them to have progeny. Subsequent to the union, the period of pregnancy and the period between the birth and the weaning of the child, when it can fend for itself, should be looked upon as sacred and during this time at least the husband and wife should scrupulously observe *brahmacharya*. But we give no thought whatever to the matter and continue to take our pleasures recklessly. Such is the sickness of our minds—a good example of incurable sickness. It is a disease which brings us to death, and until that time we wander about like insane men. It is the especial duty of married couples that they should not mistake the purpose of marriage, but should understand it aright and come together only while they have no child and desire an heir.

In our present pitiful condition, this is extremely difficult. Our diet, our way of life; our talk, the sights which surround us, are all such as to excite our lust. Sexual pleasure, moreover, has become a craving with us, much like opium. Is it likely that in such a state we would take thought and turn back? But to any sceptic who wants to know how the ideal can be practised, there is no answer in this chapter.

It is intended for those who are ready to think and make an effort to do what ought to be done. Those who are satisfied with themselves will find it boring even to read these things; the chapter is intended, rather, to help those who have realized their abject state and are tired of it to some extent.

We can see from the foregoing that those who have not married should not do so in these difficult times and that, if one cannot do altogether without marriage, one should marry late. *Young men should take a vow not to marry before they are twenty-five or thirty years of age.* This is not the place to consider the other benefits which, apart from good health, may follow from this course; everyone, however, will know how to gain such benefits for himself.

To parents who may read this chapter, we must say that they are guilty of cruelty in selling away their sons and daughters by marriage or betrothal while they are still children; in doing so, they regard their own interests instead of those of the children. They want to feel important and have a name in the community, want to have a big show by celebrating their children's marriage. If they desired the welfare of their children, they would look after their education, care for them and train their bodies. What can be more harmful to the interests of boys and girls today than that they should be married off while they are still children?

Lastly, when a married man or woman is separated from his or her partner by death, it will benefit the survivor's health to lead the life appropriate to a widower or widow. Some doctors have expressed the opinion that young men and women must have opportunities for sexual relief. There are also some others who argue that this is not necessary in any circumstances. When doctors thus quarrel among themselves, we should take care not to be misled by any of them and sink in self-indulgence in the belief that we have their support. From my own experience and that of others which I have come to know of, I can affirm without the least hesitation that it is unnecessary to indulge in sexual relations for the sake of health; on the contrary; such indulgence and the resultant loss do much physical harm. The vitality of both mind and body developed through many years is so much impaired even by one such occasion that it takes a long time to regain it and, even so, the original state is never restored wholly. One may make use of a broken glass by re-joining the fragments, but it will always remain a broken thing.

In order to conserve virility, fresh air and water, wholesome food as described earlier, and pure thought are indispensable. In this way morals are closely linked with health. A perfectly moral person alone can achieve perfect health. Anyone who, prepared to make a fresh start from the moment that he sees the light, meditates carefully over what has been said so far and puts these suggestions into practice will have direct proof in experience. Even one who has observed *brahmacharya* for some period will notice the increase of mental and physical powers and, having once secured this philosopher's stone, will guard it with care like very life. The slightest lapse and he will realize what an error he has made. I have committed mistakes even after I had thought over—experienced—the countless benefits of *brahmacharya* and I have known the bitter consequences. I have vivid memories of the exalted state of the mind before a lapse and the pitiable condition after it. But from these mistakes, I have learnt the value of that precious jewel. I do not know if I shall be able to preserve it unbroken. I hope to, with God's help. I can see the good it has done to my mind and body. I, who was married in childhood, was blinded [by lust] in childhood and had children while a mere child, awoke after many years and seem to have realized on awakening that I had been pursuing a disastrous course. If anyone learns from my mistakes and my experience and saves himself, I shall be happy to have written this chapter. The following calculation is also worth making. Many people have said, and I believe it, that I have plenty of energy. My mind is not considered weak—as a matter of fact—some think me obstinate. I have ailments of body and mind; and yet I am reckoned as fairly healthy in comparison with those with whom I have come into contact. If I have been able to maintain this condition because, after some twenty years of self-indulgence, I woke up, who can say what I would have been if I could have saved those twenty years as well. I am sure, myself, that there would have been no limit to my energy and I would have had so much of it to spend on service to the public or myself that others would have found it an ordeal to equal it. This is the conclusion to be drawn from my all-too-imperfect example. The physical, mental and moral strength of one who has been able to observe unbroken *brahmacharya* must be seen to be believed; it cannot be described.

Anyone reading this chapter will see that, when married persons have been advised to observe *brahmacharya* and widowers to continue in that state, there can be no question of any men or women, married or unmarried, being permitted to gratify their desire anywhere. It is not possible, when dealing with questions of health, to consider the dire effects of casting evil glances at other people's wives or prostitutes.

This is a matter for religion and ethics. Here, we need only state that those who indulge in such extra-marital relations and have contacts with prostitutes suffer, we find, from such unmentionable diseases as syphilis and rot away because of them. Nature is so merciful to them that it promptly incapacitates them; they keep slumbering, however, and run from doctor to doctor in search of a cure for their diseases! Where there is no adultery, fifty per cent of the doctors and *vaidyas* will lose their occupation. These diseases have such a hold on the human race that thoughtful doctors have been driven to observe that, despite all their discoveries, the nations of the world will soon be wiped out if the evil of adultery continues unchecked. The remedies for the diseases in question are so toxic in effect that, even when the diseases themselves seem to be cured, others take root in their stead and pass from generation to generation.

We shall now indicate how married couples may observe *brahmacharya* and so conclude this rather long chapter. A married person cannot observe celibacy merely by following rules regarding diet, air and water. He must also refrain from being alone with his wife. We shall realize on reflection that, except for the purpose of conjugal relations, it is not necessary to be alone with one's wife. At night the husband and the wife must sleep in separate rooms. During the day they should remain fully occupied with useful activity and pure thoughts.

They should read such books and meditate over such lives as would strengthen them in their good resolve and should frequently remind themselves that all pleasures lead to suffering. Whenever, they feel passion rising in them, they should take a cold bath. This will transform the cosmic fire in their bodies into a benign influence for both men and women and increase their happiness. All this is certainly hard of achievement, but conquering difficulties is what we are born for and. anyone who wishes to acquire good health must conquer this one.

[From Gujarati] *Indian Opinion,* 26-4-1913

NOTES

1. Literally living in the *Brahman*, the Absolute. In ordinary usage the term has come to signify celibacy, which is considered essential for attainment of that state.
2. The original has a pun on the Sanskrit word *rati* which means pleasure and, also, a measure of weight.
3. Tonic preparations of the *Unani* system of medicine behave like a dandy. *He who gives up this frame with a smiling face and goes to render his account to the Master is truly a man and she who dies thus is truly a woman.* Such persons alone may claim to have maintained true health.

18
General Knowledge About Health-XVIII

SOME REMEDIES

1. AIR

We have considered how to keep good health, on what it depends and how to conserve it. If all men always followed the rules of health and observed unbroken celibacy, the chapters that follow would not be necessary because such men cannot possibly suffer any physical or mental illness. But such persons are rare indeed. There is hardly one so fortunate as never to have fallen ill. The average person is perpetually ill with some sickness or other. Such a person will enjoy good health in the measure in which he follows the rules set out in the first part. If, moreover, he knows some simple remedies, he will not get into a panic and rush to a doctor or *hakim*[1] when he does fall ill. It is with this in mind that the chapters which follow are written.

We have seen that fresh air is the first essential for good health: it is also an invaluable cure for certain ailments. For instance, if a man whose joints have become stiff is treated with steam, there will be immediate perspiration and the joints will be relieved. This method of applying steam is known as Turkish bath.

If a person whose body is burning with high temperature is made to sleep naked in the open air, the temperature will immediately come down. He will feel easy and, if he is covered with a blanket when his body has become cool, he will begin to sweat and the fever will disappear. There is a notion among us that, when anyone has high fever, all the windows and doors should be closed, even if that should make the place unbearably hot for the patient, that the latter's head and ears should be wrapped up, and that he should be covered with heavy blankets. This is an entirely wrong notion. The practice causes the patient acute discomfort and makes him weak. It often happens that the patient, having been wrapped up in this way, perspires profusely and the thermometer shows a lower temperature, but the patient is greatly weakened. In fever brought on by heat, no one should be afraid to take the air treatment described above. The patient will immediately feel the benefit and no harm whatever will come of it. One should only make sure that the patient does not shiver when lying exposed. If he feels cold, it means that his discomfort [from heat] had not been too severe to bear after all. In case the patient is not in a condition to lie naked out of doors, there can be no harm whatever if he is made to sleep covered up in the open air.

A change of air is a highly effective remedy for prolonged fever or any other sickness. The practice of going for a change of climate is, as a matter of fact, part of the "air treatment". There is also a custom, among some, of changing houses. Many believe that a house which is never free from illness must be a haunted one. This seems to be mere superstition. The so-called haunting is in fact just polluted air. Consequently, the change of house means change of air, and that is in itself a great advantage. The air we breathe has so close a bearing on the condition of our bodies that the slightest change in it is bound to affect us for better or worse. The rich can go abroad in search of good climate. A poor man can also benefit by going to a neighbouring town or even by a change of residence. Sometimes a patient improves merely by being moved from one room to another. It is superfluous to caution here that on all such occasions the air in the room, house or town to which one goes should be better than that left behind. Sickness caused by a humid atmosphere will not disappear by a change to a more humid place. Sometimes no benefit is derived from a change of air, the reason being that the change is made without a knowledge of the principle involved. Sometimes health does not improve because, though the change has been to a better climate, other necessary precautions have not been taken, with the result that the benefit derived from a good climate is lost.

I would request the reader to compare this chapter with the one in Part I devoted to the subject of "air". The earlier chapter explained the relation between air and good health and it contained a general discussion on air. In this chapter, the therapeutic value of air is considered. Read in conjunction with this chapter, the earlier one will be better understood

[From Gujarati] *Indian Opinion,* 3-5-1913

NOTE

1. Physician practising the *Unani* system of medicine.

19
General Knowledge About Health-XIX

2. WATER TREATMENTS

Air does its work invisibly, so that we cannot fully realize the efficacy of air treatments. But the properties of water and the effects it produces are immediately apparent and we can, therefore, readily see how admirably it works.

Water treatments by steam are more or less familiar to all. We give a steam-bath to a patient suffering from fever. A bad headache can often be relieved by the use of steam. If joints are affected by rheumatism and it is desired to give the patient quick relief, treatment with steam, followed immediately by a cold bath, proves highly beneficial. When there are boils on the skin, too many of them, we cannot apply ointment or poultice to all of them, but they soften in no time if treated with steam.

When exhausted, if one takes a hot bath followed by a cold shower, one feels light in body and the fatigue disappears. If anyone suffering from insomnia takes a steam-bath, followed by a cold shower, he will, more often than not, soon fall asleep.

In most of these cases hot water can be substituted for steam. It is not necessary, therefore, to make any distinction between the two. If one suffers from stomach-ache, it can be quickly relieved by hot water fomentation. This can be done by placing a bottle or other vessel, filled with boiling water, on a cloth over the abdomen. Sometimes, it becomes necessary to cause vomiting. This can be done by drinking plenty of hot water. One suffering from constipation can get relief by drinking hot water when retiring or in the morning immediately after brushing the teeth. Sir Gordon Spring, a former Prime Minister of the Cape, enjoyed excellent health. When asked what it was chiefly due to, he replied that he drank a glass of hot water the last thing at night and the first thing in the morning. That was, he said, the secret of his good health. Some people pass a motion only after drinking tea and in their ignorance give the credit to tea. Actually the tea is harmful: it is the hot water in it that produces the effect.

There is a special kind of tub for a steam-bath, but this is not really necessary. A spirit or kerosene stove or small wood or coal fire should be placed under a cane chair or wooden stool. A pot of water should be covered and placed on the fire. A counterpane or blanket should then be spread over the chair and so arranged over the front that the patient seated on it should not feel too severely the heat from the fire or steam. The patient should be wrapped in a cotton rug or blanket and seated in the chair. The lid should then be slipped off the water pot so that the steam reaches the patient. It is our custom also to cover the latter's head but this is not necessary. Heat generated in the body rises to the head and drops of perspiration form on the face. If the patient is not in a condition to get out of the sick-bed; he may be laid on a cane couch or iron bedstead and given steam-treatment. In that case, also, the blankets should be so arranged that heat and steam do not escape. Care must be taken to see that the patient does not sustain burns and the blankets or other things do not catch fire.

Should the patient happen to be extremely weak, one should hesitate to give him steam-treatment, for if steam has its benefits, it can have harmful effects too. After taking a steam-bath, the patient always feels weak. The weakness does not last long but the treatment, if taken habitually, is bound to have an exhausting effect on the patient. Steam should, therefore, be used with great caution. It may also be applied locally. For instance, in a case of headache it is not necessary to steam the whole body. Water should be boiled in a narrow-necked vessel or kettle and the forehead held over the opening. The head should be partially covered with a cloth so that the steam may reach the head through the nostrils. If the nose is blocked, such inhalation will give immediate relief. If an inflammation is confined to a particular spot, it may be treated by applying steam to the affected part only.

The good effects of hot water and steam are fairly widely known, but few seem to know the value of cold water. To tell the truth, the beneficial properties of cold water even surpass those of hot water.

It may be said that on most people cold water has a stimulating effect. Even the weakest patient can be given cold water treatment. For fever, smallpox, rash and other skin affections, wrapping up with cotton sheets soaked in cold water is highly efficacious. The effect seems almost miraculous and anyone can test it without the slightest risk. In cases of giddiness or delirium, a piece of cloth soaked in ice-water and placed over the head gives great relief. If one has had no motion, it may be possible to get relief by applying cloth soaked in ice-cold water to the abdomen. Those who have wet dreams often get relief if they sleep every day with a cold wet bandage tied over the lower abdomen. The application of an ice pack stops bleeding in any part of the body. When the nose is bleeding, immediate stoppage is brought about by dashing a lot of very cold water on the head. One suffering from any disease of the nose, or from cold or headache derives great benefit from drawing up water through the nostrils twice a day. One nostril should be closed, water drawn in through the other and then ejected through the first. Water may also be drawn in through both the nostrils and ejected through the mouth. If the nose is otherwise clean and some of the water passes from the nostrils into the stomach, it does no harm. It is an excellent habit to clean the nose by drawing in water through the nostrils. Those who cannot manage this may do so by using a douche, but anyone can master the technique of drawing water up through the nostrils after a few attempts. Everyone should try to learn it since a headache can often be cured instantly by this easy method. If the nose gives out an offensive smell, for that, too, this is an effective remedy. Some persons suffer from a running nose; they will find the method of drawing water in through the nostrils an unfailing remedy for their condition.

Many people are reluctant to take an enema, and some even argue that it causes weakness. This is a wrong notion. There is no better method of immediate relief from constipation. In various conditions, where other remedies are ineffective, an enema provides relief. It empties the bowels completely and prevents accumulation of new poisons in the body. Anyone who suffers from gas, flatulence or any complaint brought about by poor digestion may take two pounds of water by enema, and so have an immediate rest. There is a book on this subject. Its author had tried many remedies, but failed to cure his dyspepsia. He had grown extremely weak and anaemic. With the use of the enema, his appetite improved and, in a short time he was in excellent health. Complaints like jaundice can be immediately cured by means of enemas. If this treatment has to be prolonged, it is advisable to use cold water, as hot water may cause weakness; this, however, is not to be blamed on the enema as such.

[From Gujarati] *Indian Opinion,* 10-5-1913

20
General Knowledge About Health-XX

2. WATER TREATMENTS (CONTINUED)

After numerous experiments, a German named Kuhne has discovered that certain water treatments are most effective in a number of ailments. His book on this subject has been translated into many languages. Translations are available in India also. His thesis is that the stomach is the source of all disease. If there is excessive heat in the stomach, it erupts by way of boils on the skin or rheumatism or some such trouble, or as fever, causing the whole body to become hot.

There were many before Kuhne to write on water treatments. There is a very old book called *Water Treatments*. But no one before Kuhne had laid the same emphasis as he did on the basic identity of diseases.

No one had pointed out that all ailments had their origin in the stomach. It is not necessary for us to accept Kuhne's thesis as gospel truth, nor need we go into the details of the matter. But it seems quite certain that, in a large number of cases, Kuhne's diagnosis and treatment are correct. Thousands have found this by experience. The late magistrate of Durban, Mr. Titan, was struck down by paralysis after an attack of tetanus. Having tried various treatments without success, he was advised by someone to see Kuhne. He went to him, was completely cured and lived in Durban for many years after his return.

He always advised people to try Kuhne's treatments. There is a clinic in Natal which gives his treatments. It is near Sweetwaters station. This is only one instance of its popularity; one can find many others.

Kuhne says that the excessive heat in the stomach can be removed by cooling, and for this purpose he advises a bath which will cool the stomach and the adjacent areas of the body. He has invented a special tin bath to make the process easy, but we can do without it.

Oval tin tubs of 36 inches, more or less as may suit the patient, are readily available; one of these will do for a Kuhne bath. Three quarters of the tub should be filled with cold water and the patient should be placed in it so that his feet rest outside on a board and the upper part of the trunk also remains above the water-line. Only the portion from the navel to the thigh should be submerged. The patient must be naked in water. If he feels cold, the upper part of his trunk and his feet may be covered with blankets or he or she may wear a shirt or 'a blouse, keeping it out of the water. This bath should be taken in a room which can let in light, air and sunshine and, in fact, does let them in while the bath is proceeding. After seating himself in the tub, the patient should rub his abdomen, under the water, with a rough towel or get it rubbed by an attendant. This kind of bath can be taken for 5 to 30 minutes or longer. Sometimes, the relief is immediate.

If the patient is suffering from gas, wind begins to pass or he begins to belch. If he has fever, his temperature is bound to fall by one or two degrees 5 minutes after the bath has commenced. He will have a free motion. An exhausted person will feel refreshed. One suffering from insomnia will feel relaxed and be able to sleep. One who is excessively drowsy becomes alert and lively. The reason why such seemingly opposite effects are produced has already been stated.

Lethargy and insomnia are different results produced by the same cause; they are only apparently opposites. Both diarrhoea and constipation arc similarly the results of indigestion. Some get diarrhoea while others get constipation. The bath has a highly beneficial effect on both conditions. Very old cases of piles are cured by this bath treatment in conjunction with correct dieting. If a person feels nausea, he will probably be cured immediately he starts the bath. The weak grow strong with it. Many have been cured of their rheumatism by this means. The bath is also excellent for haemorrhage and useful in cases of blood-poisoning. Anyone having a severe headache will get immediate relief with this bath. Kuhne himself thought that his baths were invaluable even in such terrible diseases as cancer. Pregnant women will have easier deliveries if they take these baths. It is a treatment that can be taken by children, by the young and the aged, by men and women.

There is another way of taking this bath which is unfailingly effective in certain ailments. It is called *the wet sheet pack*, which in Gujarati means "a bandage of wet cloth". The manner of treatment is as follows: Place a table or low seat, long enough for the patient to lie on full-length, if possible in the open air. Arrange on this four or more blankets according to the weather, so that they hang down on all sides. Spread over them two clean bed-sheets, long and thick, which have been soaked in cold water and wrung out. Place a pillow under the blankets for the head. The patient should then be stripped of all clothing, except a small handkerchief or cloth round his waist which may be retained if desired. He should be laid flat on his back between the sheets arranged as above, the arms hanging own and the [lower] sheet and blankets wrapped round him from both sides, one over the other. The covering at the bottom should be carefully wrapped round his feet. If there is sunshine, a wet cloth should be placed on his head and face, leaving the nose uncovered in all cases.

The patient will feel a momentary chill which will be immediately followed by a feeling of relief and comfortable warmth. He may remain in this condition for 5 minutes to an hour or more. By and by, the patient becomes so hot that he perspires. Frequently, he falls asleep at this stage. When he comes out of the wet sheets, he must immediately have a cold bath. This treatment is highly effective in many skin diseases. Eczema, ringworm, pimples, chickenpox, smallpox, simple boils, fever, etc., yield quickly to the "wet sheet pack". However, severe the attack, smallpox can, in most cases, be cured by this treatment. An attack of rash is cured by taking one or two baths. The technique of taking or arranging this bath is easily learnt and everyone will discover its effectiveness in experience. During the bath, the dirt from the skin is deposited on the wet sheet. The latter should, therefore, never be used again by the same or another patient until it has been thoroughly washed in boiling water.

Finally, there is one point to be kept in mind about these water treatments, that, if the bath is taken without proper attention to diet and exercise, it can never have full effect or may have no effect at all.

If a man suffering from arthritis takes the Kuhne bath or "wet sheet pack" but eats unsuitable food, does not breathe fresh air, lives in dirty surroundings and takes no exercise, he cannot hope to benefit from the treatment alone. It can be of help only if other rules of health are duly observed. There is no doubt whatever that, if they are, water treatment will help the patient to a most speedy recovery.

[From Gujarati] *Indian Opinion,* 17-5-1913

21
General Knowledge About Health-XXI

3. EARTH CURES

We have learnt something about water treatments. In some cases, earth cures, have shown even more spectacular results. Our bodies are made up largely of earth; it is, therefore, not surprising that earth should have an effect on us. All people regard earth as something sacred. The ground is coated with mud to destroy odours, earth is sprinkled over refuse, dirty hands are cleansed with earth, the private parts can also be wiped clean with earth. *Yogis* coat their bodies with mud. The original inhabitants of this country [Africa] apply mud to boils. We filter water through sand or earth in order to purify it.

Finally, dead bodies buried in earth will not pollute the air. Such, we observe, is the undoubted excellence of earth. From this we may make a fair guess that earth, probably, has some highly beneficial qualities peculiar to itself.

Just as Kuhne gave much thought to water and said many useful things about it, another German named Juste has written about earth. He goes to the extent of saying that even incurable diseases may yield to earth treatment. He reports how once, in a neighbouring village, a man bitten by a snake and even given up as dead by many was brought to him on someone's advice. Juste placed him under earth and the man soon regained consciousness. This is not an impossible thing to have happened. Juste had no reason to tell a lie. It is obvious that great heat will be generated in anyone buried under earth. We have no means of discovering how the invisible bacteria in the earth act upon the body; it does seem, however, that earth has the power to absorb poisons. By citing Juste's illustration, it is not of course intended to suggest that every case of snake-bite can be cured by earth treatment, but it should certainly be tried on such occasions. The suggestion that earth should be used for bee and scorpion stings is easier to accept. I have myself tried it on such stings and found that immediate relief followed. For this purpose, a stiff paste made of earth soaked in cold water is applied on the affected part, which is then bandaged.

The illustrations that follow are from my personal experience. A patient suffering from dysentery was cured in two or three days by the application of a mud pack to his abdomen. Immediate relief has been obtained by this method in cases of headache. Inflammation of the eyes is cured by placing a mud pack just over the affected eyes.

Swelling brought about by blows is relieved. For a number of years I could keep well only if I took fruit salt, etc. I learnt of the efficacy of earth treatment in 1904, since when I have never had to take fruit salt.

For anyone suffering from constipation, the application of mud packs to the abdomen is found to be highly beneficial. Stomach-ache also is relieved in this way. Diarrhoea can also be cured by a mud pack. High fever is reduced in an hour or two by tying mud packs to the stomach and the forehead. Boils, the itch, eczema, etc., often yield to treatment by mud pack. However, once pus is formed in the boils, mud packs are found to be of little use. In the case of burns, the immediate application of mud pack reduces pain and prevents swelling. Piles yield to the mud pack. As a result of frost, the hand and feet often become red and swollen. Mud packs are a sure remedy for this condition. Mud has been found to be good for eczema. For pain in the joints, the application of mud brings immediate relief.

From these numerous experiments with mud packs, I have come to the conclusion that as a house-hold remedy mud is invaluable.

Every kind of earth is not equally efficacious. Red earth has been found to be particularly effective. The earth to be used should always be dug out from a clean spot. Earth containing a mixture of dung, etc., should not be used. It should not be excessively sticky.

Earth which is partly sandy and partly sticky is excellent. It should be altogether free from grass or roots. It is sometimes advisable to strain the earth through a fine sieve. It must always be mixed with cold water and the paste should be of the consistency of dough. It should normally be placed in a clean unstarched piece of cloth and applied like a poultice to the affected part. The pack should be removed before the mud is about to dry up. A pack usually lasts for two or three hours. Mud from a used pack should not be used again. The cloth, however, may be used after washing, provided there was no pus on it. When mud is applied to the abdomen, a warm cloth should be placed over the pack and then the whole thing tied with a bandage.

One should have a tin of earth handy so that it can be used whenever necessary and one does not have to go hunting for it in emergency. In case of scorpion stings, etc., the earlier the mud is applied the better.

[From Gujarati] *Indian Opinion*, 24-5-1913

22
General Knowledge About Health-XXII

4. FEVER AND ITS REMEDIES

Having considered the principal remedies, we shall now turn to a few specific diseases and in the process we shall get some idea of other forms of treatment which do not call for separate chapters.

We use the term fever for any rise in body temperature but English doctors have distinguished many varieties of it and written big volumes on these, ending up in sheer confusion. As shown in these chapters, and according to the popular view of the matter, one remedy is enough for most types of fever. I have had experience of a single remedy applied in all cases of fever ranging from simple fever to the bubonic plague and I believe the results have been quite satisfactory.

In 1904, there was an epidemic of the plague among our people.[1] Twenty-three persons were attacked by it. In twenty-four hours, twenty-one cases proved fatal and only two could be removed to hospital. Of these, one survived and he happened to be the only one who could be treated with the mud pack. We cannot, of course, conclude from this that the patient was saved by the earth-treatment, but it can at any rate be maintained that the latter did him no harm.

All the victims had inflammation of the lungs and fever. They had become unconscious. A mud poultice was applied to the chest of one of them. He was bringing up blood and phlegm. After taking him to hospital, I learned from the doctor that he had previously been given very little food and that too only milk.

Fever has its origin generally in some stomach trouble. The first step to be taken therefore is fasting. The notion that a weak person or one suffering from fever will be weakened by fasting is entirely mistaken. We saw in an earlier chapter that only that food is useful which can be digested and converted into blood. The rest merely remains in the stomach like a lump of lead, as we have seen in earlier chapters. The digestive system of one who has fever becomes extremely slack. The tongue becomes dark or coated and the lips are dry.

What can a person digest in such a condition? Giving him food is bound to raise his temperature. By stopping all intake of food, we give the stomach a chance to do its work. The fast, therefore, must be continued for at least a day or longer. Kuhne baths should be administered during and after the fast. At least two should be taken every day. In the intervals between baths, a mud pack should be applied to the abdomen. If there is headache or the head feels very hot, a pack should be applied to the head also. The patient should be adequately covered but kept in the open air. The fast should be broken with orange juice added to warm or cold water. Juice should be squeezed out of the orange and strained and then hot or cold water added as required. As far as possible, sugar should not be added. This mixture of orange juice and water will have an excellent effect. If a patient can take lime juice and water without his teeth being set on edge, he should be given that. For the next meal he can take half or a whole banana, well mashed. One spoon of olive oil and half a spoon of lime juice should be added to the mashed banana and given to the patient after mixing them well. If he feels thirsty, he should be given water, which has been boiled and cooled, or lime juice and water.

Unboiled water should never be given. Cold water must always be previously boiled. Methods of purifying water have been described in an earlier chapter which should be referred to. The patient should wear only a minimum of clothing and this should be frequently changed. As he is to be covered with a sheet, very little clothing is necessary with this treatment. Some persons suffering even from such a severe illness as typhoid fever have been known to recover and, what is more, they now enjoy excellent health.

Quinine brings about an apparent cure but the patient suffers from side effects. Quinine is believed to be particularly effective for patients suffering from "malaria fever", but in fact they are rarely found to be entirely free of it, whereas I have seen even malaria patients completely cured by nature treatment.

Much reliance is placed by-others on a milk diet during fever, but my experience has been that milk taken in the early stages of fever does actual harm. It is, moreover, difficult to digest. If necessary, it should be given along with wheat, coffee or boiled with a little quantity of rice, flour and water. But in cases of obstinate or high fever, it cannot be given even in this form. At such times, I have found lime juice mixed in water to be remarkably beneficial. When the patient's tongue has become clear, the banana diet should be started, the banana being prepared in the manner described earlier. If the patient is constipated, rather than a purgative he should be given an enema of hot water mixed with borax to clear-his bowels. Olive oil in the diet will thereafter help to keep the intestines clear.

[From Gujarati] *Indian Opinion,* 31-5-1913

NOTE

1. *Vide* "Plague in Johannesburg", 9-4-1904.

23
General Knowledge About Health-XXIII

5. CONSTIPATION, SPRUE, DYSENTERY, PILES

It will certainly appear strange to most readers that four diseases are considered together in this chapter. But they are, in fact, closely related to one another and our cures for them, which require no medicines, are common to all. When the intestines are heavily loaded, some people, because of their peculiar constitution, become constipated. That is, they do not pass stools regularly and in proper quantity and have to strain. If this goes on for a long time, they begin to pass blood. This results sometimes in the rectum becoming flaccid and sometimes in piles. Still others suddenly develop diarrhoea. If the motions are numerous continuing during all hours at short intervals and in small quantities, the condition is known as sprue.

Some have dysentery in which mucus is passed and there is griping. All these patients suffer from lack of appetite, look pale, become weak, have offensive breath and a coated tongue. Some have headaches or develop other ailments. Constipation is so common that hundreds of medicines and powders have been invented for it. Mother Seagle's Syrup, fruit salt, etc., are intended chiefly to cure constipation and thousands come to harm through them, since they are apparently effective. Any ordinary *hakim* or doctor will tell us that the root cause of constipation is indigestion and will also add that constipation will disappear if the causes of indigestion are removed. The more honest among us freely admit that patients want to shake off the disease without shaking off their own bad habits, and hence, they are driven to prescribing powders and decoctions. Advertisements nowadays actually announce that those who take the medicines in question will not need to change their diet or other habits; they will be cured by the medicine alone! Those who have been following these chapters must have realized that such advertisements are fraudulent. The effect produced by a purgative is always bad. Though it may remove constipation, it will, however mild it be, give rise to other poisons in the body.

Having taken a purge, if one proceeds to change one's bad habits so that purgatives will not again be necessary, one may perhaps derive some benefit from it. Those, however, who continue with their bad habits are bound to get some other ailment even if they are cured of constipation or sprue.

We shall now consider remedies for these four diseases. The first is for the patient to reduce his diet. Heavy foods, those prepared with excessive ghee, sugar and milk kept boiling over a long time, should be eschewed. If he has any addictions like smoking, drinking, hemp-taking, etc., he must give them up. If he is in the habit of eating white bread, he should give it up. Tea, coffee and cocoa should be given up. The diet should consist mainly of fresh fruits, together with olive oil.

Treatment should begin with a 36-hour fast. During this time and later, mud packs should be applied to the abdomen on retiring and one or two Kuhne baths should be taken daily. The patient should walk at least two hours a day. Anyone following this regimen is bound to benefit. I have actually seen severe cases of diarrhoea, constipation, dysentery, and also of severe and chronic piles, cured in this way.

With regard to piles, it is necessary to insist that, as long as mucus or blood is being passed, no food is to be taken. When the patient is in a position to take food, he should have orange juice filtered and added to boiling water. In this way, the worst case of dysentery can be cured in the shortest time without harming the patient. If dysentery is accompanied by severe griping, the abdomen should be fomented with a bottle filled with very hot water or with a heated brick. As in all illnesses, the patient needs fresh air here too.

The following fruits are regarded as especially beneficial in constipation: figs, French plums, muscatel raisins, large grapes, black grapes, green grapes and oranges. One should not, however, imagine from this that these fruits should be eaten even when one is not hungry. When there is griping or a bad taste in the mouth, even these fruits can be harmful. When food is needed, these fruits will be specially beneficial in constipation, that is all that the statement above should be understood to mean.

[From Gujarati] *Indian Opinion,* 7-6-1913

24
General Knowledge About Health-XXIV

6. INFECTIOUS DISEASES: SMALLPOX-1

We have discussed a few things about fever and some other ailments. It is not intended in these chapters to go into detail with regard to all diseases. Indeed, it is unnecessary to write individually of each disease when both cause and treatment are common to all of them. Infectious diseases like smallpox also arise from the same cause and it is not really necessary, therefore, to write separately about them either. It will not be wrong, however, to devote one chapter to smallpox.

An outbreak of smallpox creates such a scare that hundreds of superstitions connected with it are current. In India, it is actually ascribed to a particular goddess and countless men and women take vows in order to be cured of the disease. Like other illnesses, smallpox arises from polluted blood, which in its turn originates in fever of the intestines. The body throws out accumulated poisons by way of eruptions. If this view is correct, there is no need whatever to be afraid of smallpox. If it was uniformly infectious, then all those who freely touch the body of the smallpox patient would catch the disease. But we know that this does not happen. There is no need, therefore, to dread smallpox, though, of course, we should take precautions against it. We cannot say definitely that it is not infectious. If anyone pre-disposed to the disease touches a smallpox patient, he will certainly get it. That is why, whenever smallpox breaks out, a number of people fall a prey to it. Because the infection is caught in this manner through contact, people are infected with cowpox and misled into believing that the cowpox infection will induce smallpox in a mild, harmless form and so prevent an actual attack of smallpox. The process consists in first infecting a cow's udder with smallpox and then introducing the vaccine taken from that part into our body through the skin, in order to induce smallpox in us and thus protect us against an attack in an acute form. At first it was believed that one vaccination of this sort would provide life-long immunity. But on experience it was found that even those who had been so vaccinated did not remain immune against infection for a very long time. It has been concluded, accordingly, that after the lapse of a certain period, it is necessary to repeat vaccination. Nowadays, the rule is to vaccinate the entire population wherever an epidemic breaks out, irrespective of whether the people had been previously vaccinated or not. One thus comes across persons who have been vaccinated five or six times or even oftener.

Vaccination seems to be a savage custom. It is one of the poisonous superstitions of our times the equal of which is not to be found even among so-called primitive societies. Its advocates are not satisfied with voluntary vaccination. They insist on making it compulsory.

Those who refuse to take it are prosecuted and awarded harsh penalties. Vaccination was invented in 1798. Thus, it is not an ancient superstition. During this short period, millions of people have been victims of it. Those who are vaccinated are presumed to be immune against smallpox, but the presumption is without any sound basis. No one can say that they would surely have had a severe attack of the disease if they had not been vaccinated. On the contrary, in view of the fact that there have been cases of vaccinated persons being attacked by smallpox, it certainly cannot be claimed that anyone getting vaccinated will escape the infection.

Vaccination is a filthy remedy. Vaccine from an infected cow is introduced into our bodies; more, even vaccine from an infected human being is used. Some persons generally vomit at the sight of the vaccine. If it so much as comes into contact with the hand, they wash the hand with soap. If we were asked to eat it, we would be nauseated and would pounce upon anyone who might make such a suggestion even in fun. And yet scarcely anyone realizes that, when he is vaccinated, he is absorbing a substance which is in reality infected blood. It is well-known that patients are given medicine or liquid nourishment through the skin and this takes effect more rapidly than if given by mouth. What is taken by the mouth is not immediately absorbed into the blood but anything taken through the skin is, and even a small dose acts very quickly. From this point of view, the taking of any medicine or nourishment through the skin is the same as eating it.

Even then, in order to save ourselves from smallpox, we, in effect, eat vaccine. It is said cowards die before their death. Similarly, from fear of death or disfigurement by smallpox, we die before our time by getting ourselves vaccinated.

I personally feel that in taking this vaccine we are guilty of a sacrilege. Even meat-eaters are forbidden to drink blood, and the flesh and blood of living animals are, I find, prohibited in all circumstances.

But here blood is taken from a blameless living creature, is cultured, besides, and then fed to us through our skins. A religious man would rather get smallpox a thousand times or an early death than take such blood.

[From Gujarati] *Indian Opinion,* 14-6-1913

25
General Knowledge About Health-XXV

6. INFECTIOUS DISEASES (CONTINUED): SMALLPOX-2

A number of thoughtful men in England have carried out researches on the harmful effects of vaccination and a big anti-vaccination society has been formed. Its members refuse vaccination and oppose the law making it compulsory. Some have suffered imprisonment in this cause. They also advise others against vaccination. Many books have been written on the subject and much discussion is being carried on. The following are the reasons the opponents of vaccination advance in support of their stand:

1. Taking vaccine from a cow's udder, which in fact belongs to her calf, is itself an act of extreme cruelty to thousands of living creatures. This cruelty is no credit to man's sense of pity and it behoves him, therefore, to forgo any benefit that may accrue from it.
2. No benefit is derived from such vaccine. On the contrary, taking the vaccine causes other infections. The sponsors of this movement are of the opinion that, since vaccination was introduced, the incidence of other diseases has increased.
3. The infection originates in man's blood, so that the germs of other diseases in the person are likely to be present in the culture and in all the samples of the vaccine.
4. Vaccination does not guarantee protection from smallpox. Its inventor, Dr. Jenner, had claimed that

vaccination at one spot on one arm would provide life-long immunity. Later, he said vaccination on both arms would give such immunity. Then, it came to vaccination on more than one spot on both arms. When the disease occurred in spite of this, it was said that immunity could not be guaranteed for more than seven years. This period has now been reduced to three years. Thus, doctors themselves are far from certain in this regard. In fact, the idea that one who is vaccinated will never get smallpox is entirely untrue. No one can prove that a person who has been vaccinated and has never caught smallpox would have caught the infection if he had not been so vaccinated.

5. Finally, they hold that vaccination is a filthy practice and that it is sheer barbarism to imagine that filth can be removed by filth.

With these and many other arguments and illustrations, the anti-vaccination society has been able to exert a great influence on the British public. There is a town in England where the majority of the population refuse to be vaccinated and, yet, the incidence of the disease among them is very low. Some enthusiastic members of this society have probed carefully into the whole question and have shown that doctors find it in their interest to keep this superstition alive. They earn thousands of pounds annually through vaccination. Consequently, either intentionally or otherwise, they are blind to its harmful effects. This opinion has been expressed by certain doctors themselves and most of these have strongly opposed vaccination.

If, then, vaccination is harmful, should we submit to it? My personal reply would be a definite "No". There are certain exceptions, however. I am certain that no one should get himself vaccinated voluntarily. But in all places where we have settled, the law has made vaccination compulsory. In this country ([South] Africa), to break the law involves a tremendous risk, for, if we refuse to comply with it, we shall invite on ourselves the charge of wilfully endangering public health, in addition to the many other charges often made against us.

What should we do in such circumstances? If we live where the majority believe in the benefits of vaccination, it becomes something of a duty for us to fall in line with them to avoid a panic among them.

Those who object to vaccination on religious grounds, in view of the facts I have set out above, must resist it even if they have to stand alone and must be prepared to suffer the consequences. Those who refuse vaccination merely in the belief that they would remain healthier on that account would not be justified in opposing the law in this regard outright. Anyone who wants to do so must have made a thorough study of the matter. He should be able to convert others to his point of view and should undertake to change public opinion. If one cannot do these things, one may not ignore public opinion merely to protect one's health. There are many things which we dislike and yet feel compelled to do out of regard for the society in which we live. Personal convenience has to yield to public interest.

The accepted principle is that only in matters of morality or religion do situations arise in which a man will be justified in standing alone against the opinion of the majority. Those, however, who have no belief of their own but are possibly swayed by writings such as the present one and are unwilling to be vaccinated through sheer apathy, should certainly abide by the law.

Further, those who do not get vaccinated must take pains to study and observe the rules of cleanliness, etc. One who does not want smallpox infection [by way of vaccination] and, at the same time, contracts diseases on account of immoral conduct or suffers in other ways by disregarding the rules of hygiene, has no right to oppose vaccination in a country or society in which it is regarded as a means of preserving health.

[From Gujarati] *Indian Opinion,* 21-6-1913

26
General Knowledge About Health-XXVI

6. INFECTIOUS DISEASES (CONTINUED): SMALLPOX-3

Writing of smallpox, we have so far considered the harmful effects of vaccination. We must now study ways of preventing smallpox.

One who faithfully and intelligently observes the rules concerning fresh air, water and diet described in earlier chapters is in no danger of getting smallpox because his blood will itself contain the antidote against the infection.

For one who has contracted the disease, the wet sheet pack is a miraculous remedy. The pack should be applied to the patient at least three times. This will reduce the burning sensation in the body and the sores will subside in a very short time. It is not necessary to apply ointment, etc., to the sores. If the latter are limited to one or two spots where mud packs can be applied, that also should be done. The patient should be given rice, lemons and light fresh fruit according to appetite. I have said "light fruit" because, when the body is burning with smallpox, highly nourishing fruit such as dates and almonds should not be eaten. The sores are bound to subside after a week's treatment with the wet sheet pack. If they do not, it means that some poison still remains in the body and is being thrown out. Smallpox need not be regarded as so very serious a disease. It is only a symptom of poison escaping from the body and, therefore, of the body regaining health.

The last explanation applies to many diseases but is more likely to be correct in regard to diseases of the smallpox group.

The reason why some patients remain weak or suffer from other ailments, after recovery, is to be found not in the original disease but in the remedies employed. Thus, quinine taken for malaria often causes deafness.

Some even get a serious complaint known as quininism. Venereal diseases are cured with mercury, etc. The disorders which this gives rise to, as is well known, remain with the patient forever. Thus, medicines not only do not cure the disease but in fact cause new ones.

We shall find numerous instances of patients who resort to purgatives in order to cure constipation and develop piles, etc., in consequence. To understand and remove the basic cause of a disease and, when the latter has disappeared, to obey the laws of Nature is a better tonic than any *bhasma*[1]. Metals are processed so as to make them assimilable and turned into powders like *lohabhasma*[2]. But it is wrong to regard these as unfailing remedies. They do indeed seem to have some beneficial properties, but to the extent that they benefit the body, they strengthen the passions. Thus, they are ultimately harmful to one in their total effect. These medicines find greater favour as cures for smallpox. One who has had an attack of this disease rarely contracts it again. As a matter of fact, he often enjoys excellent health after his recovery because all poisons from the body have been drained out.

When the attack subsides and the sores dry up, olive oil should be applied to the skin and the patient regularly bathed. If this is done, most of the scars will disappear altogether and new skin will be formed.

[From Gujarati] *Indian Opinion,* 28-6-1913

NOTES

1. Form of metallic medication in *Ayurveda.*
2. *Bhasma* with properties of iron.

27

General Knowledge About Health-XXVII

7. OTHER INFECTIOUS DISEASES

We have considered smallpox in some detail. Now remain allied diseases such as chickenpox, measles, etc. The plague, cholera, and fast-spreading dysentery are also infectious diseases. We are not afraid of chickenpox and measles because they are seldom fatal, nor do they cause disfigurement. Apart from this, they are very similar in effect to smallpox and are contracted in the same manner. Cold water treatments and wet sheet packs are the best remedies for them. Diet during the attacks should be extremely light and bland. If a patient can subsist on fresh fruit, his recovery will be rapid.

The "tumour fever" is a terrible disease. In English it is called "the bubonic plague". Hundreds of thousands have died of it in India since 1896. Despite much fuss, doctors have so far been able to discover no remedy for it. Now-a-days, a preventive inoculation similar to vaccination is given for this disease also. Producing with it a mild attack of the plague, the doctors explain that this will confer immunity against further infection. But this is a mockery similar to vaccination and is an equally sinful experiment. Just as it cannot definitely be stated of anyone who has been vaccinated that he would surely have got smallpox if he had not been vaccinated, so also is it impossible to say that one who has been inoculated against the plague would have got it were it not for the inoculation. There is no known antidote against the bubonic plague. Nor can any guarantee be given that water and mud treatments will prove effective against the disease. However, for the benefit of those who do not fear death and who have trust in God, the following measures may be suggested:

1. On getting fever or at the very first signs of it, take a wet sheet pack.
2. A thick mud pack should be applied to the swollen glands.
3. The patient should be given no food whatever.
4. If he feels very thirsty, cold lime juice and water should be administered.
5. The patient should lie in a place open to plenty of fresh air.
6. Except for one person, no one should be allowed to go near him.
7. If anything can bring about a cure, these measures certainly will.

No definite knowledge is available regarding the origin of the plague. Many, however, are of the opinion that it is spread by rats and there seems to be some basis for this impression. In areas where cases of the plague have occurred, it is imperative that houses be cleared of rats, and that grains, etc., be stored so that rats cannot gain access to them and are not attracted. Rat-holes should be filled in; if a house cannot be completely freed of rats, it must, of course, be vacated.

But the best insurance against the plague is to adopt from the start a clean, wholesome and spare diet, give up all addictions, take regular exercise, live in fresh air, keep one's home and surroundings clean and thus maintain oneself so fit that this fashion of a plague does not touch one. This should be the normal manner of living but, even if that is not possible, it should in any case be followed while an epidemic is on.

An even more terrible disease and one which breaks out simultaneously with the bubonic plague is fever accompanied by difficult breathing, known in English as the pneumonic plague. The temperature shoots up very high and the patient remains for the most part unconscious. Recovery from this *kalajwar*[1] is rare. This disease came to Johannesburg in 1904 and only one out of twenty-three cases survived. Some account of this incident has already been given. For this condition, too, the remedies are the same as those suggested for the bubonic plague, except that in this case it is necessary to apply mud packs to both sides of the chest. If there is not enough time in which to keep the patient in a wet sheet pack, thin mud poultices should be applied to the head. For this disease also preventive Cholera appears horrible when there is an actual case but, in fact, it is a much less serious disease than the plague. Wet sheet packs cannot be used here because the patient suffers from cramps, especially in the thighs. It may be of some benefit in this condition to apply mud packs to the abdomen, but where there are cramps it is necessary to foment the spot with hot water bottles. The patient's feet should be rubbed with mustard oil. No food, of course, must be given.

The patient's friends should see that, instead of his getting scared out of his wits, his courage is kept up. If he has frequent motions, he should not be made to leave bed for the purpose, but he should be provided with a shallow pan without sharp edges in which he may pass stools. If these measures are taken without delay, there will be little risk for the patient. During an epidemic of cholera, there are effective measures with which to protect oneself against it. The disease usually appears in summer. People suddenly start eating unripe or rotten fruit.

We are not as a rule accustomed to eat fruit, but many kinds ripen in this season and are cheap, so that they are eaten in large quantities. This is in addition to the usual food, with the result that the harmful effect of such fruit follows immediately. Even as it is, we frequently suffer from stomach-ache and such other complaints. When the stomach can stand the strain no longer, we get cholera. Others' physical condition is similar to ours and hence they also get an attack.

No special precautions are taken regarding the patient's stools and the germs from these pollute the atmosphere. Water also is bad during the hot weather. With everything going dry, water becomes dirty and infected and is drunk without being filtered or boiled. Under such conditions, is it any wonder that diseases occur? It is only because Nature has provided us with a tough physique that we survive at all.

Otherwise, looking at our conduct and habits, we deserve a very early end indeed. We shall now consider the precautions to be taken during an epidemic of cholera. It is very important to keep the diet light and moderate. Good fruit may certainly be eaten but it should be carefully examined. We should never, out of miserliness or because of their tastefulness, eat mangoes or any other fruits which are rotten in parts.

Fresh air is essential. *Drinking water must always be boiled* and filtered through a thick and clean piece of *khadi*[2]. Excreta of patients must be burned and the place covered with dry earth. If it became a regular practice with every person to sprinkle ashes over the excreta after using the latrine, the danger would be greatly reduced. To tell the truth, this should be a permanent rule. Cats dig a hole into which they pass stools and then cover it up with earth. It is only we who neglect to do this, thinking it to be a kind of pollution or feeling squeamish about doing it, and so fall victims to disease. If ashes are not available, dry earth should be used. If in lumps, the earth should first be broken up and made into dust.

The fast-spreading dysentery is the least serious of these infectious diseases. In this condition, if only mud packs are properly applied to the abdomen and all intake of food stopped, the disease will be cured. It is essential that excreta be covered up in the manner described above. In regard to water, the same precautions should be taken as for cholera.

Finally, when any of these infectious diseases occurs, neither the patient nor his friends and relatives should lose courage. With fear, the patient will succumb much sooner, and his relatives, and others as well, will be in danger of catching the infection.

[From Gujarati] *Indian Opinion,* 5-7-1913

NOTES

1. Literally, deadly fever measures are easier to take and more effective than remedies for cure, and it will be wise to employ these as shown an page 100.
2. Any coarse cloth; later, in India, the term came to signify hand spun and hand woven indigenous cloth.

28
General Knowledge About Health-XXVIII

8. CONFINEMENT

We have so far considered general diseases. It is not the intention, in these chapters, to write on all the maladies one may come across in this world or make suggestions about them, but rather to show that most diseases have a common origin and a common form of treatment. Those who have been driven to desperation by illness and are afraid of death will certainly consult a doctor, whatever books are placed before them. The most that these chapters can indicate is how those who suffer from ordinary ailments may recover and, observing the laws of good health, may not fall ill again or become a prey to a serious disease. Only a few have the courage even for this.

That those few may find these brief articles useful is one of the objects in view in the present series. We have now reached a point when, after a brief consideration of confinement, infant-care and accidents, we may conclude these chapters.

The subject of confinement has been made too much of. Delivery is nothing very dangerous for a woman whose body is healthy.

Among villagers, a confinement is regarded as a very ordinary occurrence.

Pregnant women perform their usual tasks right up to the last and suffer no harm during child-birth. There have been cases of *Bharwad*[1] women resuming normal work immediately after giving birth to a child. Animals, we know, suffer no pain.

Then, why do urban women suffer so much pain? Why do

they suffer such unbearable agony during the birth of a child? Why does it become necessary to give these women special care before and after delivery? Let us take up these questions.

The city women's way of life is completely unnatural. Their diet and dress are opposed to Nature's laws. The most important. reason, however, is something quite different. If a girl becomes pregnant while she is still a child, if her husband does not refrain from intercourse with her even during this period and, soon after delivery, so conducts himself that within a short time she becomes pregnant again, why will she not suffer? We see hundreds of thousands of girls and women in this fearful and pitiable condition. City-life of this kind is no different from hell. As long as men continue thus to behave like monsters, women can never be happy. Many men blame women. It is not our business in this chapter to say who is more to blame. Whether it be the fault of both parties or of one, having realized that something is wrong, parents, child husbands and child-wives should take heed. As long as intercourse during childhood, during pregnancy and immediately following confinement is not given up, deliveries can never be easy. Because the women do not have to suffer excessively for a very long period and as it is considered inevitable that they will be weak for a month and a half afterwards, they put up with the ordinary pains of child-birth and, thanks to the prevailing ignorance about this state of affairs, a race of cowardly, emasculated and spiritless creatures is coming into existence day by day. This is a terrible thing indeed, and each one of us needs to work tirelessly to prevent it. If even one man or woman shuns such evil practice, that will be so much gain to the whole world. In this matter, one should never wait for another to make a beginning.

According to this view, then, the first step to be taken in the care of a pregnant woman is for her husband to stop all sexual intercourse with her. Many responsibilities are to devolve upon her during the nine months of pregnancy. It should be realized that the future conduct of the child will depend to a great extent upon that of the mother during this period. If the mother is affectionate, so will the child be. If she is bad-tempered, the child too will be bad-tempered. It is quite important, therefore, that the mother should maintain a very pure state of mind during these nine months. She should be engaged in virtuous deeds, avoid anger, be particularly compassionate and generous, be free from anxiety and fear, not allow carnal thoughts even to enter her mind, not waste time in useless gossiping, and never tell an untruth. If a woman observes all these rules, the child to be born to her cannot but grow to be an illustrious person.

Just as it is imperative that the mind be kept pure, so also must the body be kept clean. It is essential always to have fresh air. During pregnancy, the woman's respiration becomes more rapid. Consequently, she must be in a place where the air is much fresher. Her diet should be regular, easy to digest and nourishing. A good diet should be planned along the lines recommended in earlier chapters. She should consume during this period olive oil, bananas and wheat in quantities which she can digest. If she gets constipated, she should not go in for any medicine but increase the quantity of olive oil. If suffering from nausea, she should take lime juice in a little water without sugar. Spices, chillies, etc., should be completely stopped, during these nine months, at any rate.

Some women feel all kinds of fanciful desires and aversions at this time. The best way to combat them is to have regular Kuhne baths. This bath will increase strength, improve the lustre of the skin and ensure easy delivery. Many women have had this experience. It is also necessary to control these fancies when they come. It is possible to forget an object which the mind hankers after by disregarding the desire on one or two occasions. At all times, both mother and father must be careful of the safety of the child she is carrying.

It is the husband's duty not to agitate the wife by starting quarrels with her during this period. She should be kept happy and relaxed. If she has to carry too heavy a burden of domestic work, the husband should try to lighten it. It is essential for her to have a short walk in the open air every day. During pregnancy, it should be seen to it that no medicine of any kind is swallowed by the mother.

[From Gujarati] *Indian Opinion*, 12-7-1913

NOTE

1. A Community of shepherds in Gujarat.

29
General Knowledge About Health-XXIX

9. CARE OF CHILDREN

It is not intended in this article to go into the details with which midwives are concerned. We shall therefore, turn to the time after the child has been delivered. Those who have understood the previous chapters will realize that even during confinement it is not necessary that the mother and child must be kept roasting in a dark, unventilated room, with bedding all too dirty and heated from beneath. However, old the practice of keeping a confined woman in a dark room, it is cruel all the same. Keeping out fresh air is even more cruel. The custom of placing fire under [the cot] is entirely unnecessary and one full of risk. During the winter the patient will certainly need greater warmth. For this purpose, she should be supplied with extra coverings.

If the room is cold, a fire, first lighted outside, may be brought in after the smoke has subsided, and the air in the room be warmed but it is absolutely unnecessary to place it under the cot. A hot water bottle in the mother's bed will as well help to keep it warm. It is also a cruel and superstitious practice to provide her with dirty sheets to sleep on. After recovery, the clothes can be thoroughly washed and used again. The child's health depends on the condition of the mother.

Therefore, in addition to these precautions, she should be given an easily digestible and nourishing diet. There is no evidence that [tonic foods made with] gum and things of that kind are particularly beneficial. If the mother eats a diet of wheat, banana and olive oil, sufficient heat will be generated in her body and she will have plentiful supply of milk. Olive oil will give milk a mildly laxative quality, and this will ensure clear motions for the child. If the baby has any complaint, it is the mother who should be examined. To give any drug to the baby will be risking its life. The child's intestines being extremely delicate, the toxic effects of the drug will be felt immediately. At such times, it is the mother who should take the medicine as its curative properties will in an imperceptible manner pass into her milk. If the baby appears to have too many motions or to be coughing frequently, there is no need for panic. Instead, one should wait for a day or two. The specific cause of the trouble should be removed and the child will recover. Flying into a panic and giving medicines will definitely harm the baby's health.

Infants should be bathed in lukewarm water and should have a minimum of clothing. For the first few months it will be better for the baby to have no clothing at all. It is best wrapped in a soft white sheet and then covered with a warm shawl. In this way the bother of dressing the child is avoided. Fewer clothes will be soiled and the baby will come to have a tough rather than a weak constitution. A folded thin cloth should be laid over the umbilicus and a bandage tied over it. The custom of tying the umbilical cord to the neck with a string is bad. The bandage should be changed every day. If there is any raw skin round the umbilicus, finely strained powder of cleaned rice should be sprinkled over it with clean cotton wool. This will help the part to dry up.

As long as the mother has a plentiful supply of milk, it is unnecessary to give the infant any other food. When the supply decreases, the child should be given the flour of roasted wheat, mixed with warm water and a little jaggery and this will have the qualities of milk. Alternatively, half a banana mashed and well mixed with half a spoon of olive oil will prove very beneficial. If cow's milk is to be given to start with, a mixture of one part milk and three parts water, heated to boiling point, should be used. A little quantity of pure jaggery should also be added to this. Substituting sugar for jaggery seems to be harmful. If the child is gradually given increasing quantities of fresh fruits, its blood will remain in excellent condition from the very start and it will grow strong and vigorous. Many mothers feed babies with *dal*, rice, vegetables, etc., as soon as its teeth appear or even earlier than that. But this is undoubtedly no good for it. Tea and coffee should in no case be given to a child.

When the baby has grown up, that is, has learnt to walk, it may be dressed in a shirt, etc. Shoes are quite superfluous. An infant does not have to walk among thorns. If, therefore, it remains barefoot, the child's feet will be toughened and there will be no obstacle to the circulation of blood which might otherwise be constricted because of the shoes. It is both vulgar and cruel to dress up a child, for the sake of show, with silken clothes, or dresses padded with cotton, narrow *pyjama*, a cap on head and ornaments round the neck. To imagine that we can improve upon the appearance that Nature has given the child is sheer vanity and ignorance.

It must be realized that the child's education begins right from its birth and that its real teachers are its father and mother. To threaten a child, to pad its body [with dresses], to overload its stomach all these are a violation of educational principles. If the parents are irritable, the child will grow likewise, and from parents who are soft it will learn to be soft. Its ways of speech also it will learn from the parents; if the parents pronounce words correctly, so will the child; if they use stammering or foul speech, the child will do likewise. If they follow immoral ways, to be sure, the child will learn them. "As the father so will be the child, as the banyan tree so will be its fruit"[1]—is indeed a true saying. Here, the word 'father' stands for both parents. The child learns to eat the food the father eats. Later on, it will never get elsewhere the education that it can receive in its home.

When we consider all this, it becomes clear how very delicate is the responsibility the parents carry. Man's primary duty is to teach children purity of conduct so that they may bring credit to themselves and the parents. We observe of trees and their fruits that only plantains can come from a plantain tree and that an excellent tree alone produces good fruit. A fine animal has fine offspring. Man falsifies this rule. Parents with a reputation for purity have children of impure conduct and apparently healthy parents have unhealthy offspring.

The chief or rather the only reason for this is that, though not worthy to be parents, we frequently become such merely in consequence of self-indulgence. How then can we be mindful of children's interests? But it is incumbent on right-minded parents to bring up their children in the best possible manner. To be able to do this, both father and mother must have received true education. Parents who have not done so should, if they realize their error, leave their children in the charge of other well-educated and virtuous persons. It is vain to hope that children will learn good behaviour at school. There is only one way of teaching good behaviour and that is to give the child an opportunity to live constantly in that kind of atmosphere. If there is one sort of training at home and another at school, the children can never improve. It follows from this that there are no fixed times when a child is to receive its education. Its education commences at its birth and from that very moment begins its physical, mental and spiritual or religious training. Its training in language starts the moment it begins to prattle. Instruction in letters also it can have from its parents, as it plays. In olden days, this was what usually happened. Now, it has become the custom to send children to schools. If parents would do their duty by their children, there would be no limit to the heights the latter could reach. But, if we regard children merely as toys, fondle them excessively, spoil them out of a mistaken notion of affection with sweets and rich clothes right from their childhood, allow them to do as they please, if we are greedy for money ourselves and teach this greed to children, are engrossed in pleasures and set that example before children, are lazy ourselves and make them lazy, are dirty and teach them dirty ways, tell lies and teach them lies, then is it any wonder that our progeny grow up to be feeble, immoral, lying, lustful, selfish and greedy? Thoughtful parents need carefully to ponder over these remarks. India's future, a good half of it, lies in the hands of parents.

[From Gujarati] *Indian Opinion*, 19-7-1913

NOTE

1. A Gujarati saying.

30
General Knowledge About Health-XXX

10. ACCIDENTS: DROWNING

We have made a brief study of certain ailments. Everyone should have some knowledge regarding accidents that may occur at any time so that he can render assistance if anyone is in mortal danger. If children are given such knowledge from quite an early age, they are likely to develop kindliness in greater measure.

We shall begin with the treatment to be given to one who may have fallen into water. In England, a philanthropic association has been established to render assistance in such emergencies. It has issued some valuable suggestions. The following note is chiefly based on these, with some modifications and additions. It is said that a person can live for hardly five minutes after he stops breathing. That means that, when a drowning man is taken out of the water, there is little life left in him. Immediate measures have to be taken to keep life going—to bring the drowning person back to consciousness. Two things must especially be attended to in such a case. One is to make the victim resume normal breathing by giving artificial respiration and the second is to give him warmth. When thinking of remedies, it has to be kept in mind that immediate treatment has to be given, if needed, at places like river banks where no equipment is available. It is possible to render treatment to a drowning man only if there are two or three other persons present. These must possess presence of mind, courage and promptness. If they themselves fall into a panic, nothing can be done. If each of the two or three men wants to follow his own method or starts advising the others, there is little hope for the victim. They must immediately recognize the most capable among themselves and follow his instructions at once.

As soon as the victim is taken out of the water, his wet clothes should be removed. His body should be wiped with any cloth the companions may have. A hand should then be placed on his forehead and he should be gently turned over for a minute. A hand should be pressed against his chest and dirt and water removed from his mouth.

When the tongue comes out, it should be held. This can be easily done with a handkerchief, etc., kept ready in the hand. The tongue should be kept pulled out all the time, till there are signs that life is reviving.

The patient should then be turned on his back, but with the head and upper parts a little higher than the feet. A man should now kneel behind his head. The patients' arms should be slowly lifted and drawn full length towards the person volunteering this service. With this the ribs will be lifted and air from without will enter the patient's body.

Then the arms should be bent and placed on his chest. Thereby, the ribs will be pressed down and the breath exhaled. Hot and cold water should be dashed against the chest. If the materials required to make a fire are within reach or if fire can be obtained immediately from some source, fomentation should be applied and the victim be made warm.

Those present should cover him with whatever clothes they have. His body should be vigorously rubbed so as to make it warm. It is necessary to continue these measures for quite some time. Hope should not be abandoned too soon. Dr. Moore states that with these measures a victim resumed breathing even after five hours. They should be taken, therefore, with great energy and promptness. If he comes round, the patient should be given a hot drink. If given orange juice in hot water or a decoction of cinnamon, cloves and pepper, he will quickly rally. It may also help if he is made to smell tobacco.

People should not crowd round him as he has need of all the fresh air he can get. Signs of death in these cases are generally as follows:

The victim does not breathe and no heart-beat can be detected by the hand or stethoscope. There is no pulse, the eyes are half closed, the pupils are dilated, the jaws are clenched, the fingers are bent, the tongue is between the teeth, there is froth in the mouth, the nose is slimy and the whole body extremely pale. A feather held over the mouth does not flutter nor does vapour collect on the mirror. If all these symptoms are present, it may be taken that life is extinct. But Dr. Moore says that even with these signs, life is sometimes not over. The only definite symptom of death is that decomposition starts within the body. We may conclude from this that hope should be abandoned only after prolonged treatment has been given.

[From Gujarati] *Indian Opinion,* 26-7-1913

31
General Knowledge About Health-XXXI

11. ACCIDENTS: BURNS

When any person's clothing or something else about him catches fire[1], we get into a panic, which is like branding a man who has already sustained burns[2]—instead of being helpful to the victim, we make things worse for him. It is everyone's duty therefore to know what remedies to apply to a man who has suffered burns.

The person whose clothes catch fire should also not become terrified but, if it is the loose end of a garment, should promptly rub it with the hand. If the entire clothing has caught fire, he should roll on the ground or, if there is a carpet or similar thick cloth within reach, he should wrap himself in it. If water is available, it should be thrown on the flames. As soon as the fire is extinguished, he should be examined for burns. If there are any, the cloth is likely to stick to those parts. This should not be pulled off. The remaining clothing should be cut round with a pair of scissors and the part that has stuck to the skin left in place. Great care should be taken not to tear the skin. Leaving the victim in this condition, one should collect clean earth forthwith and mix it with cold water to make a poultice and this should be tied over the burns so that the victim will suffer the minimum of pain. If cloth is sticking to the burns, it may safely be left under the bandage. As soon as the mud dries, the poultice should be changed. There is no need to be afraid of using cold water.

For anyone who may not think of this treatment at the

moment, here are others which will be useful to note. They are taken from a book by a British writer. Take a green banana leaf and spread olive oil or sweet oil [sesame oil] over it]. Then place it over the burn and tie it up. In the absence of a leaf, a clean soft cloth soaked in oil will do as well. A mixture of linseed oil and lime water in equal proportion and well shaken is also effective. If cloth pieces get stuck and cannot later be removed, lukewarm milk and water should be used to soak them.

When they are softened, it will be possible to remove them. If oil bandages have been used, they should be changed after two days in the first instance and subsequently renewed every day. If a blister is formed, it is necessary to open it. The skin need not be removed. If the burn has only caused redness of the skin, there is no better remedy than a mud poultice. The burning will cease immediately.

If the fingers have been burnt, they should be kept carefully separated from each other by clean bandages. Sometimes, a person receives burns through a strong acid which falls on his skin. The remedies suggested above are effective in this case also.

[From Gujarati] *Indian Opinion,* 2-8-1913

NOTES

1. "Brother"; this was how associates addressed Gandhiji.
2. A Gujarati saying.

32
General Knowledge About Health-XXXII

12. ACCIDENTS: SNAKE-BITE

Men have always feared snakes. There are countless superstitions, too, connected with the serpent. We are afraid even to mention its name. At night we refer to it as "the big creature". Among Hindus, the snake is an object of worship. *Nagpanchami*[1] is regarded especially as the day of snake worship. There is a popular belief that the earth is supported on the head of the serpent *Sheshnag*. God also is held to be *Sheshshayi,* i.e., lying on *Sheshnag*. God Shiva is said to wear a snake as a garland. "*Sheshnag* with his thousand mouths could not describe this"; in saying this we attribute intelligence and knowledge to the serpent. There is a similar idea in Christianity also.

"Be wise as the serpent", so runs a saying in English. The serpent *karkotak* conferred a boon upon Nala[2] by biting him, thereby making him so ugly and deformed through its poison, that none would look upon him with evil intent as he wandered in the forests. The serpent also stands, in the Bible, for the Devil. It was he who tempted Eve.

Thus, there are all kinds of beliefs and tales about this creature. It is easy to understand the dread of snakes. If a snake-bite takes full effect, death is inevitable, and no one wishes to die. Hence, this fear. It is also easy to see how snakes have been worshipped out of fear. If the snake had been a tiny creature, it would not perhaps have inspired such worship despite its being the terror that it is. But being long, large, beautiful and of strange aspect, it is even ceremonially worshipped.

It is more difficult to say without thinking why the snake has been credited with intelligence. Modern scientists aver that it has none.

According to them, a snake should be killed at sight. Government statistics show that in India 20,000 people perish annually from snake-bite. I think the figure must be higher. The Government offers a reward for every poisonous snake killed; it is doubtful, however, if the offer has served any useful purpose. This confirms the general experience that the snake does not bite without cause. It bites only if attacked or teased. Does this possibly indicate intelligence, or, if not that, harmlessness? It uses its fangs in its own defence. Man also uses teeth for that purpose often enough. To attempt to make India or any other place entirely free of snakes is like trying to wrestle with the air.

Snakes can be prevented from coming to a particular spot. Killing the ones found entering the place will prevent others. They will come to realize that going to the place is like walking into the jaws of death. But this can be done only for a limited area. The attempt cannot be made over a vast country like India. To seek, therefore, to kill and extirpate the snakes entirely in this way from the country amounts to throwing money down the drain.

Moreover, it is the same God who creates snakes [as well as ourselves]. We cannot understand all the works of God. Surely, he has not created beings like tigers, lions, snakes and scorpions only so that we may kill them! If the snakes themselves were to get together and consider how men killed them at sight, they would ask if God had created man for the sole purpose of destroying them. Just as that would be a mistaken belief, so would be ours regarding snakes.

St. Francis was a great *Yogi* in Europe. He used to wander in the forests among reptiles, etc., but they never harmed him. On the contrary, they were friends with him. Thousands of *Jogis*[3] and *fakirs* live in the forests of India. They move fearlessly among tigers, wolves, snakes, etc., and one never hears of their coming to any harm on that account. It might be argued that there must be casualties even among them through snake-bites, or predatory animals; this is very likely. We know, though, that in comparison with the great number of reptiles, etc., the *jogis* and *fakirs* are so few that if these deadly creatures, were set on destroying them, not one of them would survive. We are told—and we believe it to be true—that these *jogis* and *fakirs* keep no weapons with which to withstand these beasts. This proves that some dreaded beasts are friendly to or, at any rate, do not touch some *Jogis* and *fakirs*. I personally feel that when we rid ourselves of all enmity towards any living creatures, the latter also cease to regard us with hate. Compassion or love is man's greatest excellence. Without this he cannot cultivate love of God. We come to realize in all the religions, more or less clearly, that compassion is the root of the higher life.

Furthermore, is it not possible that the very existence of creatures like snakes or the cruelty in their nature reflects our own attitudes?

Is there not cruelty enough in man? On our tongues there is always poison similar to a snake's. We tear our brethren to pieces as wolves and tigers do. Religious books tell us that when man becomes pure in heart, the lamb and the tiger will live like friends. So long as in our own selves there is conflict between the tiger and the lamb, is it any wonder that there should be a similar conflict in this world-body?

We but mirror the world. All the tendencies present in the outer world are to be found in the world of our body. If we could change ourselves, the tendencies in the world would also change. As a man changes his own nature, so does the attitude of the world change towards him. This is the divine mystery supreme. A wonderful thing it is and the source of our happiness. We need not wait to see what others do.

The purpose of writing at such length on the subject of snake-bite is that if, instead of merely suggesting a few concrete remedies, we go deeper into the matter, we discover a miraculous remedy with which to face all such terrors and, if even one reader adopts it, my writing this will not have been in vain. It has been said earlier, moreover, that the purpose of these chapters on health is not merely to promote physical health but examine the means of cultivating health of every kind.

Even modern research-workers admit that a man who is healthy, whose blood is not overheated and whose food is wholesome, will not be affected by snake venom. On the other hand, if a man's blood is overheated with intoxicants, spices, or hot foods, snake venom spreads through his body in no time and he succumbs to it quickly. All this has been experimentally established by medical experts. One of them has gone so far as to declare that the blood of a person who discards salt and lives exclusively on fruits becomes so pure that it is able to combat poison of any kind. It is not possible to confirm from experience how far this last statement is true. Moreover, having abstained from salt, etc., for a year or two, one is not justified in believing that the blood which had lost its quality through a life-time's abuse had regained it because of wholesome living for a year or two.

It has also been demonstrated through experiments that if any poison gets into the system of one who is nervous or in a rage, the effect is instantaneous and more potent. Everyone can discover for himself that, when frightened or angered, the pulse is faster and the heart-beats increase. Whenever, the blood circulates at a greater speed, it becomes hot. Heat generated by anger, etc., is unnatural and, therefore, deleterious. There is no reason to doubt that rage is a kind of fever. We can at least infer from this that one of the best defences against snake-bite is to have only as much as we need of wholesome food, that is, food which Nature has placed at our disposal, to avoid anger and fear and, even when bitten by a snake, not to fall dead with fear before even a remedy has been tried. One should have confidence in the potent effect of the purity of one's life and ultimately take courage in the thought that the length of one's days is that ordained by God.

That many deaths which are apparently due to snake-bite are in reality caused by fear or wrong treatment has been confirmed by Mr. Fitz-Simon, head of the museum in Port Elizabeth. He has studied snakes for many years and performed experiments on their poison.

He has written much about the different types of snakes and also suggested remedies for their bites. He states that he has known cases where the condition had become serious owing to sheer panic and others where the persons had died as a result of extremely painful remedies.

All snakes are not poisonous and even the venom of those that are does not cause instantaneous death. Moreover, the most poisonous snake does not always get time to empty the entire poison from its fangs into our blood. Knowing this, no person need be terrified by a snake-bite. An easy remedy is current nowadays which one can apply oneself. This is as follows:

> A handkerchief should be bound tightly just above the spot where one has been bitten by the snake. This can be tightened by means of a tourniquet made with a pencil or piece of stick. The idea is to prevent the venom from circulating through the arteries. Then a cut should be made, half an inch in size, over the bite with a fine blade and allowed to bleed. After this, the purple powder of a salt called potassium permanganate should be rubbed into the cut. This powder is said to be a potent and unfailing remedy. A tube about one and a half inches in size and shaped like a stick, with facility for holding the potassium permanganate on one side and with a small, sharp blade on the other, is also available in the market for one shilling. If this implement is not at hand, either another person or the victim himself should suck the wound and spit out the matter he has sucked up. This cannot be done by anyone who has sores in the mouth as the sucked-up matter contains poison. This method is effective only if it is employed within five to seven minutes of the bite. Once, the poison has entered the blood stream, it is rarely that it can be neutralized.

Juste, who has experimented with mud treatment, declares that he cured a patient who was supposed to have succumbed to a snake-bite.

The victim was placed in a hole dug in the earth and given warmth; the poison was drawn out, and there he was, rising again. Juste reports other similar instances. I have no personal experience of snake-bite but, having tried the mud treatment in many other cases, I have come to have unshakeable faith in it. Immediately, after a cut has been made at the spot where the bite has occurred and potassium permanganate rubbed in, or the poison sucked out, a large mud poultice, half an inch thick, should be placed over it. For instance, if the hand has been bitten, it would be well to cover the entire arm with the poultice.

Everyone should keep a tin of such earth ready in his house. It will be excellent if the earth be ready powdered and strained, and better still if kept outside in the sun, at a level where water cannot reach it.

Bandages made from torn clothes should be kept handy. These preparations prove useful not only in cases of snake-bite, but also for other accidents, injuries, etc.

If the patient feels drowsy or his breathing stops, artificial respiration, as in the case of drowning, should be given. In the former case, he should be given warm water or a decoction of cloves and cinnamon. The victim should be kept in the open air but well covered.

If his body is getting cold, hot water bottles should be placed round his body or he should be warmed with the help of flannel pieces wrung out in hot water.

[From Gujarati] *Indian Opinion*, 9-8-1913

NOTES

1. Fifth day of the bright half of *Bhadrapad*.
2. A victim of the Kalipurusha, the malignant spirit of the Iron Age, he lost his kingdom and was cruelly separated from his wife, Damayanti. The story is told in the *Mahabharata* for the benefit of Yudhishthira.
3. Corrupt form of *Yogi*, used commonly for ascetic.

33

General Knowledge About Health-XXXIII

CONCLUSION

These chapters on the subject of health have been appearing for the past few months. They have now come to an end. If I get time, I plan to publish, as a sort of supplement, the qualities and uses of a number of simple materials. The present series, however, ends with the preceding chapter. Before I take-leave of my readers, I feel it will not be out of place if we once again examine the purpose of these chapters.

I have repeatedly asked myself why I wrote them. I am not a *vaidya*. My knowledge of the subject is but superficial. Is it not likely that my suggestions have been made after inadequate thought or observation? In truth, both study and observation are bound to be incomplete, a process without end. Everyday new facts are observed and new ideas emerge. Why, then, this effort? Thus, has my mind been perplexed.

And yet, medical science is itself based on inconclusive experiments. Most of it is quackery, as I have shown. With so much of it about, if these chapters are also reckoned as such, no great harm will be done! They have been written from a worthy motive. The intention is not to recommend what medicines to take after the onset of a disease. The more immediate purpose, rather, has been to show how sickness may be averted. A little thought will show that the steps for prevention of diseases are easy enough. No specialized knowledge is necessary for this. The difficulty lies in taking to that way of life. I have felt it proper to write on certain diseases, but only in order to show that most ailments have a common origin and, as a result, the treatment also should be common to them all. Moreover, despite all precautions, the diseases mentioned in these chapters do occasionally occur. Some remedies for these, one finds, are known to all. If my experience is added to these, nothing is likely to be lost.

The main question, however, still remains to be considered. Why is good health necessary? We behave as if no such necessity exists. To be sure, rather than build a stout and healthy body and give it over to the enjoyment of luxuries, regard the body as the only thing worth preserving and be puffed up with pride to see it strong, it will be better to have it rotting with leprosy.

All religions have looked upon this body as a place where one may meet and recognize God. It is called the House of the Lord. It has been leased to us, all the rent we have to pay being praises of the Master. Another condition in the rent note is that we must not misuse it. It should be kept clean and pure inside and out and returned to the Master in due course in the same condition in which it came to us. If all the conditions are duly fulfilled, the Master will reward us at the end of our tenure and will make us his heirs.

All living creatures have bodies alike in their design, in that they have organs for hearing, sight, smell and pleasure. But the human body has been described in prose and verse as a *Ratnachintamani.* The term signifies a jewel which secures to one anything one may wish for.

In an animal body, the soul cannot attain to the highest knowledge and cultivate devotion to God. Without these, there can be no freedom for the soul and, so long as the soul has not attained freedom, there can be no true happiness and no ending to our real suffering. This body is of some service only if it is well used, that is, made the abode of God, otherwise, it is a filthy mass of bones, flesh and blood, and the breath and water that exude from it are full of poison. Of all the excreta coming out of the innumerable openings in the body, there is nothing that we would wish to retain. One is nauseated at the very thought or sight or touch of them. It is only with the greatest difficulty that we can prevent them from being infested with worms.

By means of the body, we practise a thousand things which we would do better to avoid, cunning, self-indulgence, deceit, stealing, adultery, etc. Its desires are endless.[1] Even when they are all gratified, it is so like a glass bangle that it has less strength to resist a blow than has a broken vessel. It is destroyed in an instant.

Such a state is quite natural for the body. Anything that can be used for the highest purpose is also capable of being misused.

God is striving for mastery over the body, and so is Satan engaged in a desperate struggle for it. When it is under the control of God, it is like a jewel. When it passes into the control of the Devil, it is a pit of filth. If engrossed in pleasure, gorging itself the whole day with all variety of putrifying food, exuding evil odours, with limbs employed in thieving, the tongue uttering unworthy words and taking in unwholesome things, the ears hearing, the eyes seeing and the nose smelling what they ought not to, the body is worse than hell. Everyone recognizes hell for what it is. But though we use the body as if it were hell, we go on pretending that it is heaven. Such is our hypocrisy in regard to the body. Knowing a latrine for what it is, we shall know its right use. If a splendid hall, however, comes to be used as a lavatory, the result is bound to be evil. Therefore, if the body be in the Devil's control, it would be far better to desire its destruction, rather than its well-being.

In these chapters on health, an effort has been made to bring home the truth that the body can remain in health only by obeying the laws of God. It can never be healthy if it the Devil. Where there is real health, there alone is true happiness possible, and in order to achieve real health we must conquer the palate. If we succeed in this, all other organs will be automatically under our control and one who has this body under control can subdue the world because such a one becomes God's heir, a part of Him. Rama is not in the *Ramayana,* nor Krishna in the *Gita. Khuda* is not in the *Koran*, nor Christ in the *Bible.*

They all live and have their being in the purity of human conduct, which springs from morality. Morality consists in truth, which is the same as *Shiva*[2]. You may know it by whatever name you please. That one may have a glimpse, if only occasional, of this truth in these chapters on health has been the underlying purpose of this effort.

[From Gujarati] *Indian Opinion,* 16-8-1913

NOTES

1. The original Gujarati saying literally means: "That little pot must needs have thirteen things." Otherwise, it would be impossible to know or estimate its value. We can measure the value of sunlight because we experience the darkness that follows the Sun's absence. In that same Sun, without which we cannot live, resides the power to turn us to ashes. A king can be both magnanimous and wicked.
2. God of austerity and self-mastery in the Hindu trinity.

Index

Absurdity, 61
Accidents, 7, 103, 110, 113, 115, 120
Aching feet, 61
Acid content, 48
Addictions, 33, 36, 89, 100
Adultery, 29, 69, 123
Agakhan Palace, 50
Aged person, 12
Agriculture, 54
Ailments, 5, 8, 32, 44, 46, 48, 51, 56, 59, 69, 71, 78, 80, 88–89, 91
    common, 7
    ordinary, 103
Air
    bad, 15
    change of, 72
    cold, 19
    defiled, 20
    fouled, 13
    good, 63
    inhaled, 12
    insufficient, 21
    open, 59, 71–72, 80, 86, 105, 120
    polluted, 72
    pure, 14, 20
    raw, 20
    spewed, 14
    treatments, 72, 74
Airborne germs, 47
Alcohol, 32–33
    addict, 32
Allied diseases, 99
Almonds, 39, 48–49, 97
Antidote, 97, 99
Anti-vaccination society, 94–95
Apathy, 96
Aphrodisiacs, 64
Appetite, 77, 88, 97
Arctic regions, 38
Army camps, 24
Arogya Samrakshan Shastra, 1
Asphyxiation, 21
Asthma, 46
Astronomy, 55

Bad temper, 9
Bandage, 19, 84, 107, 113, 120
    cold wet, 76
Barbarism, 95
Bath, 79–81, 86, 105
    cold, 70, 74, 80
    hot, 74
    special tin, 79
    treatment, 79
Battersea Municipality, 36
Beasts, 28, 117
    dreaded, 117
    non-carnivorous, 39
    predacious, 39
Belief, 4, 8, 34, 68, 96, 115–16
    common, 8
    popular, 115

Birds cluster, 55
Blindness, 66
Blood-poisoning, 79
Body temperature, 85
Bowels, 65, 77, 87
Brahmacharya, 63–66, 68–69
Breathing, 19–20, 100
Bronchial tubes, 11
Burning sensation, 97
Burns, 83, 113–14

Cane chair, 75
Cane couch, 75
Carelessness, 23
Celibacy, 69
Chickenpox, 80, 99
Child-birth, 103–4
Child-care, 7
Child husbands, 66, 104
Child-wives, 66, 104
Cholera, 99, 101–2
Christianity, 115
Cinnamon, 111, 120
City-dweller, 21, 55
Clean bandages, 114
Cleanliness, 24, 96
Cleansing process, 4
Cocoa plantations, 36
Coffee, 32, 34–37, 87, 89, 108
Coffee lovers, 36
Cold shower, 74
Cold water, 3, 76–77, 79–80, 83–84, 86, 111, 113
Cold water treatments, 99
Community dinners, 51
Confinement, 103–4, 106
Constipation, 25, 74, 76, 79, 83, 88–90
Coriander, 45
Cotton rug, 75
Cow, 47
    diseased, 47
    healthy, 47
    infected, 92
    tuberculous, 47
Cowpox infection, 92

Death
    early, 93
    fear of, 9, 93
    instantaneous, 118
    troubled, 5
Diarrhoea, 79, 83, 88–89
Diet
    banana, 87
    ideal, 40, 50
    light, 102
    minimum, 51
    non-vegetarian, 48
    nourishing, 106
    saltless, 46
    vegetable, 42
    vegetarian, 42, 48
Digestion, 34, 45, 52, 77
    aid, 28
    salt stimulates, 46
Digestive
    powers, 35
    process, 11, 46
    system, 86
Discomfort, 72
Dishes
    special, 30
    spicy, 45
Divine
    anger, 66
    mystery, 117
Drowsy, 79, 120
Drug advertisements, 6
Dust particles, 19, 25
Dysentery, 83, 88–89
Dyspepsia, 43, 77

Earth treatment, 7, 82–83, 85
Eczema, 80, 83
Educational principles, 108
Enema, 76–77, 87

Epidemic, 6, 85, 92, 100
European
  dress, 61
  travellers, 38
Evil
  intent, 115
  practice, 104
Exaggeration, 25
Extra-marital relations, 69

Famine-stricken, 14
Fascination, 8
Fasting, 52, 86
Fever
  high, 72, 83, 87
  malaria, 87
  prolonged, 72
  tumour, 99
  typhoid, 86
Flatulence, 51, 77
Food
  chief, 38
  cooked, 42
  digest, 11
  intake of, 86, 102
  over-spicy, 45
  pungent, 45
  putrifying, 123
  spewed, 14
  sweet, 49
  tasty, 29
  unsuitable, 51, 81
  vegetable, 39
Foul
  air, 14–15, 20
  odour, 16
  speech, 108
Fresh air, 5, 10, 13–15, 20–22, 40, 57, 68, 71, 81, 89, 97, 100, 102, 105–6, 111
Fruits, 27, 39–40, 42, 48, 66, 89–90, 101–2, 108, 118
  citrus, 40
  diet, 40, 42, 48
  dry, 39, 48
  nourishing, 97
  rotten, 101
  strength-giving, 48
  sun-ripened, 39
Fruit salt, 6, 52, 83, 88

Ghee, 43, 48
Ginger juice, 36
God Shiva, 115
Gospel truth, 78
Green vegetables, 46
Grind wheat, 43

Haemorrhage, 79
Hakim, 4–5, 15, 71, 88
Hand mill, 43
Hawkers, 56
Headaches, 61, 75–76, 83, 86, 88
Heart-beats, 112, 118
Heavy foods, 89
Hiccups, 51
Hospitality, 33, 51
Hot water, 47, 74–77, 87, 111, 120
  bottles, 101, 106, 120
  fomentation, 74
Hunger, 28, 31
Hygiene, 1, 14, 30, 96
Hypocrisy, 64, 123
Hypocritical nature, 30

Ice pack, 76
Ice-water, 76
Ill-effects, 26, 46, 48
Illness
  mental, 71
  severe, 86
  slightest, 4
Immoral conduct, 96
Imprisonment, 94
Indentured labour, 36
Indigestion, 43, 57–58, 79, 88
Inexorable laws, 30
Infant-care, 103

Infatuation, 64
Infectious diseases, 91, 94, 97, 99, 102
Inflammation, 75, 83, 85
Insomnia, 74, 79
Intercourse, 104
Intestines, 11, 32, 39, 87–88, 91
Intoxicants, 35, 117
Intoxication, 34
Invisible bacteria, 82

Kleptomania, 9

Laxative effect, 43
Lethargy, 79
Lime juice, 86–87, 105
Lord Curzon, 35
Lungs, 10–16, 19–20, 85

Measles, 99
Meat, 38, 48, 93
Mental
  activity, 54
  development, 56
  energy, 40
  fitness, 34
Milk, 27, 35, 37, 42–43, 47–49, 85, 87, 89, 107
  cow's, 47, 107
  diet, 87
  lukewarm, 114
  products, 48
  woman's, 47
Mother Seagle's Syrup, 88
Mud
  packs, 83, 85–86, 89, 97, 101–2
  poultice, 85, 114
  treatments, 99, 119

Negroes, 38, 45
Non-vegetarian elements, 48
Nose smelling, 123
Nostrils, 12, 51, 75–76
Nourishment, 12–13, 27, 35, 40, 51, 93
Nutritive elements, 42

Odour, 61
  bad, 9, 51
  offensive, 61
Oil, 48, 114
  bandages, 114
  linseed, 114
  mustard, 101
  olive, 40, 47–49, 87, 89, 98, 105–7, 114
  sesame, 114
Opium, 33, 67
Orange juice, 86, 89
Organic forms, 46

Pain, 4–5, 8, 83, 96, 103, 113
  ordinary, 104
  suppress, 4
Panic, 71, 96, 107, 110, 113
  sheer, 118
Patients
  malaria, 87
  smallpox, 91
  tuberculosis, 15, 17
Permanent teeth, 11
Philanthropic association, 110
Physical activity, 57
Piles, 46, 79, 83, 88–89, 98
  chronic, 89
Pimples, 51, 80
Plague, 2, 20, 85, 99–101
  bubonic, 85, 99–101
  pneumonic, 100
Predatory animals, 116
Purity of mind, 9

Radical improvement, 61
Rain water, 25
Religious
  principle, 38
  training, 109
Respiration, 13
  artificial, 110, 120

Rheumatism, 48, 74, 78–79
Roman Catholics, 52
Rules of hygiene, 14, 96
Running nose, 76

Sexual
 pleasure, 67
 relations, 68
 relief, 67
Skin diseases, 80
Slavery, 29–30, 48
Slovenliness, 20
Smallpox, 76, 80, 91–99
Snake
 bite, 83, 115–20
 venom, 117
 worship, 115
Staple diet, 20, 39
Steam-bath, 74–75
Stomach-ache, 74, 83, 101
Suffocation, 14
Superstitions, 4, 20, 47, 72, 91, 95, 115
 ancient, 92
 sheer, 4
Superstitious practice, 106

Tastefulness, 102
Tea, 28, 32, 34–37, 75, 89, 108
 habit, 35
 merchants, 35
Therapeutic value, 73
Tobacco, 32–34
Tonic foods, 106
Toxic substances, 12
Tuberculosis, 15, 20–21
Turkish bath, 71
Typhoid, 23, 47

Umbilical cord, 107
Unnatural thirst, 26
Unshakeable faith, 119

Vaccination, 92, 94–96, 99
 effects of, 94, 97
 voluntary, 92
Vaidya, 4–5, 15, 57–58, 69, 121
Venereal diseases, 98
Venom, 46, 118–19
Vomit, 14, 28, 52, 92

Water
 bad, 23, 26
 boiling, 25, 37, 74, 80, 89
 brackish, 25
 -closets, modern, 16
 distilled, 25
 drinking, 14, 24–25, 102
 filter, 82
 foul, 14
 hard, 25
 ice-cold, 76
 lime, 114
 lukewarm, 107
 opium, 33
 polluted, 14, 23
 pot, 75
 pure, 10, 25
 soft, 25
 treatments, 74, 78, 81–82
 wheel, 30
White flour, 42